ANGELA S.

Radiographic Procedures:
a Pocket Index

For Elsevier:

Commissioning Editor: Dinah Thom
Development Editor: Catherine Jackson
Project Manager: Gail Wright
Senior Designer: Sarah Russell
Illustration Manager: Merlyn Harvey
Illustrator: Cactus Design

Radiographic Procedures: a Pocket Index

Alanah Kirby MSc DCR(R) FHEA

Senior Lecturer, School of Health Sciences, Queen Margaret University, Edinburgh, UK

Margaret Cockbain BA DCR(R) PGCertMammography

Lecturer, School of Health Sciences, Queen Margaret University, Edinburgh, UK

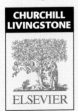

CHURCHILL LIVINGSTONE

ELSEVIER

EDINBURGH LONDON NEW YORK OXFORD PHILADELPHIA ST LOUIS SYDNEY TORONTO 2008

CHURCHILL
LIVINGSTONE
ELSEVIER

First published 2008

ISBN 978-0-443-10177-9

British Library Cataloguing in Publication Data
A catalogue record for this book is available from the British Library

Library of Congress Cataloging in Publication Data
A catalog record for this book is available from the Library of Congress

Note

Knowledge and best practice in this field are constantly changing. As new research and experience broaden our knowledge, changes in practice, treatment and drug therapy may become necessary or appropriate. Readers are advised to check the most current information provided (i) on procedures featured or (ii) by the manufacturer of each product to be administered, to verify the recommended dose or formula, the method and duration of administration, and contraindications. It is the responsibility of the practitioner, relying on their own experience and knowledge of the patient, to make diagnoses, to determine dosages and the best treatment for each individual patient, and to take all appropriate safety precautions. To the fullest extent of the law, neither the Publisher nor the Authors assumes any liability for any injury and/or damage to persons or property arising out or related to any use of the material contained in this book.

The Publisher

ELSEVIER your source for books,
journals and multimedia
in the health sciences

www.elsevierhealth.com

Working together to grow
libraries in developing countries
www.elsevier.com | www.bookaid.org | www.sabre.org

ELSEVIER | BOOK AID International | Sabre Foundation

The
publisher's
policy is to use
**paper manufactured
from sustainable forests**

Printed in China

Contents

Preface

The rationale behind this book was to provide a quick reference to plain radiological examinations and commonly performed contrast studies, together with current thinking on the imaging requirements for particular pathologies.

It is assumed that the reader already has sufficient knowledge of the basic principles of radiographic positioning and terminology and so these details are not repeated for each investigation. Rather, a reminder of general patient position, part position, tube angulation and centring point is provided. To aid in this, a selection of diagrams provide visual assistance with patient position, surface anatomy and three-dimensional planes of the body.

Each radiology department will have different imaging equipment, protocols and exposure factors of which the radiographer/ student radiographer must be aware. The aim of this book is not to be prescriptive but to aid decision-making by providing information on the advantages and relevance of each technique and by indicating any additional modalities currently used. The format of the index therefore includes basic projections, alternative projections, additional projections and alternative/additional modalities.

The first-post diagnostic radiographer is expected to perform not only plain radiographic examinations but also many contrast studies, either in the radiology department or in the operating theatre. Although many are being replaced by alternative modalities, the most commonly performed are included in this index.

The additional sections continue to provide information to aid the decision-making process. The first delineates the properties of the various contrast media in use and the second provides an explanation of the possible effects of irradiating a fetus and the rules for radiation protection of women of childbearing age. These are both areas where an understanding of the concepts is much more useful than merely memorised protocols. Some surface dose reference levels are also provided for quick comparison.

A detailed grasp of anatomical, physiological, pathological and radiological terminology is required by the radiographer or student radiographer; rather than include an exhaustive list of terminology to be read and remembered, an index of the roots of medical terms has been added. By using these prefixes and suffixes to trace the derivation of an unknown word, not only will its meaning be revealed, but deeper understanding achieved.

A common problem for student radiographers or new radiographers is that of becoming familiar with the vast array of abbreviations or shorthand notations used by the various health professionals in different departments and so a list comprising the most commonly used clinical terms has been provided.

This book is aimed at radiography students and newly qualified radiographers, and complements the more detailed and illustrated radiographic technique books on the market. The size of the book will allow it to be carried in the pocket of a uniform without hindrance in a clinical environment. The alphabetical presentation is intended to offer a speedy search facility, with cross-referencing to related techniques.

Alanah Kirby
Margaret Cockbain

Edinburgh 2007

SECTION 1

Introduction to positioning

Anatomical planes

Sagittal plane   Any vertical plane passing through the body which separates it into right and left sections. The median sagittal plane or mid-sagittal plane (MSP) separates the body into right and left halves.

Coronal plane   Any vertical plane passing through the body which separates it into anterior and posterior sections. These planes lie at 90° to the median sagittal plane.

Transverse plane   Any plane which divides the body into superior and inferior sections. These can also be called axial planes and divide the body into horizontal cross-sections.

Relative terms

Anterior	Towards the front of the body. Can also be called ventral.
Posterior	Towards the back of the body. Can also be called dorsal.
Superior	Towards the head. Can also be called cranial or cephalic (cephalad).
Inferior	Towards the feet. Can also be called caudal (caudad).
Medial	Towards the midline of the body.
Lateral	Towards the side of the body.
Proximal	Towards the origin of the structure.
Distal	Away from the origin of the structure.
Oblique	Rotation of the body from the anatomical position in either direction.

Movements

Flexion	Bending of a joint to approximate the components.
Extension	Stretching out of a joint to elongate the components.
Internal rotation	Pivot towards the centre of the body.
External rotation	Pivot away from the centre of the body.
Supination	Move to lie with anterior surface upwards.
Pronation	Move to lie with anterior surface downwards.
Adduction	Move limb towards the centre of the body.
Abduction	Move limb away from the centre of the body.
Elevation	Raise to create an angle with the horizontal.
Inversion	Rotate towards the midline.
Eversion	Rotate away from the midline.
Decubitus	Description of patient position when using a horizontal beam.

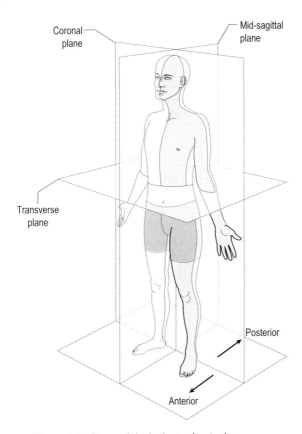

Figure 1.1 Planes of the body standing in the anatomical position

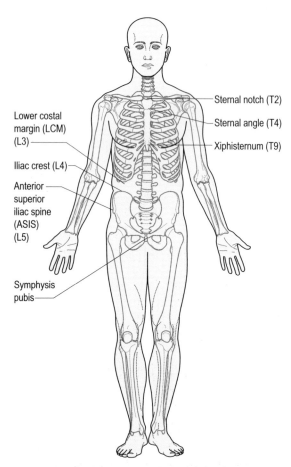

Figure 1.2 Surface anatomy of the anterior aspect of the body

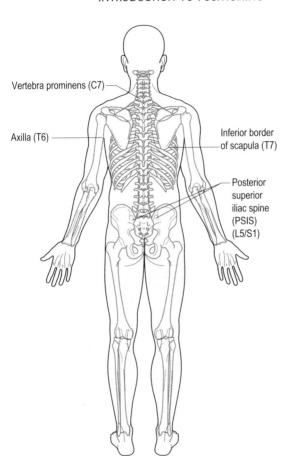

Vertebra prominens (C7)

Axilla (T6)

Inferior border of scapula (T7)

Posterior superior iliac spine (PSIS) (L5/S1)

Figure 1.3 Surface anatomy of the posterior aspect of the body

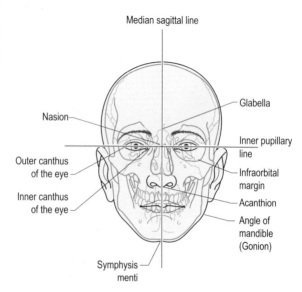

Figure 1.4 Surface anatomy, lines and planes of the skull (frontal)

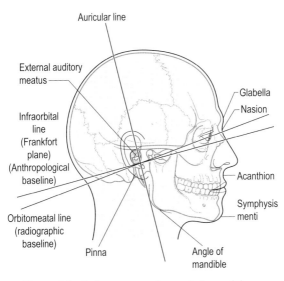

Figure 1.5 Surface anatomy, lines and planes of the skull (lateral)

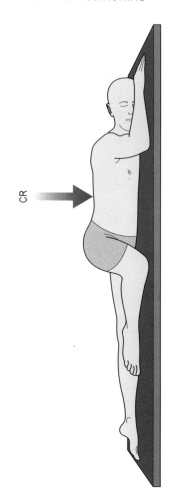

CR

Figure 1.6 Left anterior oblique position (prone)

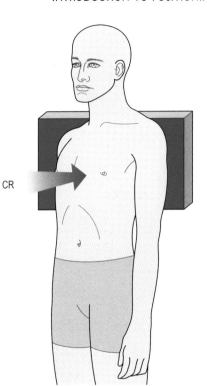

CR

Figure 1.7 Right posterior oblique position (erect)

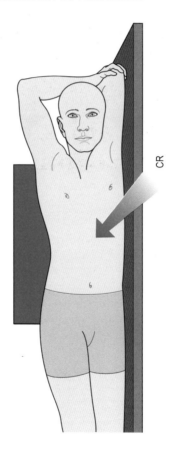

CR

Figure 1.8 Left lateral decubitus position

SECTION 2

Index of radiographic examinations

Radiographic examinations

- A source to image distance (SID) of 100 cm and a central ray (CR) at 90° to the image receptor (IR) should be assumed for all projections unless otherwise stated.
- Appropriate orientation of the IR is assumed, e.g. long axis of long bone/limb to long axis of IR.
- For projections of the axial skeleton and abdomen, anteroposterior (AP)/ posteroanterior (PA), pelvis and abdomen, the mid-sagittal plane (MSP) should be perpendicular to the IR and the coronal plane parallel to the IR.
- For lateral projections of the axial skeleton, the MSP should be parallel to the IR and the coronal plane perpendicular to the IR.
- Appropriate use should be made of anatomical and procedural markers, collimation and radiation protection measures.
- Immobilisation devices may be employed where appropriate and necessary.
- Infection control procedures should be observed at all times.
- Relevant patient preparation is assumed, including removal of potential artefacts from the region of interest (ROI).

Abdomen (*see also* Biliary tract; Diaphragm; Foreign bodies; Intravenous urography)

Basic projection

To demonstrate soft-tissue structures, calcifications, bowel gas and foreign bodies. Also used as a preliminary investigation to other imaging procedures. *BROAD FOCUS*

AP *FFD 100cm   35 X 43 1R lengthways in bucky or grid.*
- Patient supine.
- Centre to midline at the level of the iliac crests.
- Exposure on arrested expiration (inspiration will ensure that the diaphragm and symphysis pubis are demonstrated on a single exposure but the image should be labelled accordingly).
- Gonad protection can be used on males.
- Women of childbearing age should comply with local rules regarding radiation protection.

Additional projection

To demonstrate calcification of the aorta and blood vessels, an aortic aneurysm or abdominal masses. *BROAD FOCUS.*

100cm
Lateral abdomen   *35 X 43 1R lengthways in bucky or grid.*
- Patient in true lateral position with hips and shoulders superimposed.

INDEX OF RADIOGRAPHIC EXAMINATIONS

- Raise arms above head.
- Flex knees.
- Centre along mid-axillary (coronal) plane of patient at the level of the iliac crest.
- Exposure on arrested full expiration.

Additional projection

To detect imperforate anus in infants.

Ventral decubitus (lateral)
- The patient should lie prone with the pelvis over a supporting pad for at least 10 minutes prior to this projection being performed.
- IR positioned parallel to the MSP at the level of the pelvis.
- Centre to the IR with a horizontal beam.

NB: An anatomical marker should be fixed in position on the skin over the usual site of the anus. This allows preoperative measurement of the distance between the skin surface and the distal bowel, which should be delineated with gas in this position.

Additional projection

To demonstrate any free fluid or air under the diaphragm which may indicate alimentary perforation, bowel obstruction or a subphrenic abscess in acute patients.

Erect AP

- The patient should be erect for at least 5 minutes prior to exposure to allow time for any free gas to settle under the diaphragm.
- Patient seated with legs apart or standing with back towards an erect grid device.
- Centre a horizontal beam to the MSP at the level of the lower costal margin.
- Exposure on arrested respiration.

NB: This projection is now rarely used, an erect chest projection having replaced it in the Royal College of Radiologists' (RCR) guidelines for imaging the acute abdomen.

Alternative projection

To demonstrate fluid levels or free intraperitoneal air in the abdomen in patients unable to achieve an erect position. It is preferable to carry out a left lateral decubitus to avoid any confusion between gas in the fundus of the stomach and free air in the abdomen.

Lateral decubitus (AP)

- Patient should lie on their left side for at least 5 minutes prior to this projection being performed.

- Elevate patient on radiolucent pads.
- Raise arms above head and flex knees for stability.
- Place patient close to edge of couch with back in close contact with grid device (patient safety is a priority).
- Centre to midline with a horizontal central ray at the level of the iliac crests.
- Exposure on arrested full expiration.

Alternative projection

For patients unable to be moved into the lateral decubitus position.

Dorsal decubitus (lateral)

- Supine patient positioned against an erect grid with arms raised.
- Flex knees.
- If necessary, elevate patient on radiolucent pads.
- Centre a horizontal beam to the mid-axillary plane at the level of the iliac crests.
- Exposure on arrested respiration.

Additional modalities

- Ultrasound may be used as the first option in some paediatric patients.

- Computed tomography (CT) may provide more detailed information on the site and extent of any urinary obstruction.
- Radionuclide imaging (RNI) may be used to demonstrate renal function.

Acetabulum (see *also* Hip; Pelvis)

Right and left posterior oblique projections (Judet views) are used to accurately locate acetabular fractures following an AP projection of the pelvis.

Basic projections

Internal oblique
- Patient in the 45° posterior oblique position with the affected side raised.
- Centre to a point 5 cm inferior to the anterior superior iliac spine of the affected side.
- Demonstrates the posterior rim of the acetabulum.

External oblique
- Patient in the 45° posterior oblique position with the affected side down.

- Centre to the symphysis pubis.
- Demonstrates the anterior rim of the acetabulum.

Additional modality

- CT may provide reconstructed three-dimensional images for better preoperative planning.

Acromioclavicular joint (see *also* Shoulder)

To demonstrate subluxation of the acromioclavicular joint.

Basic projection

AP oblique

- Patient in the AP erect position.
- Rotate body 10° laterally to bring the shoulder of the affected side against the IR.
- Arms relaxed by the sides.
- Centre 1 cm above the head of the humerus.
- Exposure on arrested respiration.
- The normal shoulder exposure should be reduced by approximately 7 kVp.

NB: The contralateral view, taken for comparison, is no longer recommended as routine in IR(ME)R 2000. If both joints must be examined, they should be imaged separately to avoid including the highly radiosensitive thyroid gland in the field of view.

NB: By placing a weight in each hand (e.g. sandbag, water-filled bottle) for a few minutes prior to exposure, it was thought that small acromioclavicular separations could be better visualised. However, this practice is now in question.

Acromion process (see Shoulder)

Ankle

Basic projections

To indicate bony injury to the lower tibia, fibula and talus. *FINE FOCUS*

AP 18×24CM 100FFD

- Patient supine/seated with the affected ankle resting on the IR.
- Foot dorsiflexed to avoid superimposition of the calcaneum on the joint space.

- Lower limb internally rotated to bring the malleoli equidistant from the IR.
- Centre midway between the malleoli.

100cm   Fine Focus   18×24cm

Lateral

- Patient rotated to the affected side.
- Dorsiflex the foot.
- Knee flexed and supported on a pad.
- Ankle resting on the IR with malleoli superimposed.
- Centre to the medial malleolus.
- Collimation to include the head of the 5th metatarsal.

Additional projection

A fracture of the distal tibia or fibula could indicate a proximal contra-coup fracture at the proximal portion of either bone and projections of the whole tibia and fibula should be acquired if this is suspected.

- *See* Tibia; Fibula.

Additional projections

To demonstrate torn lateral/medial ligaments.

Stress projections
- AP projections whilst the radiologist or orthopaedic surgeon inverts/everts the ankle.

NB: Radiation protection issues for staff must be considered if the patient is held in position.

Alimentary tract (see Barium studies; Foreign bodies)

Aorta (abdominal) (see also Abdomen)

Additional modalities

- Ultrasound (US) is the modality of choice to demonstrate an aortic aneurysm as, unless there is associated calcification, plain radiography is equivocal.
- CT is used for detailed assessment of the extent of, and relationships to, the aneurysm.

Aorta (thoracic) (see Chest)

Arthrography

Arthrography can be described as the direct injection of contrast agent(s) into the capsule of a joint to demonstrate its internal soft tissue anatomy. Single or double contrast techniques can be used. Single contrast studies utilise a water-soluble iodinated contrast agent, the amount required varying with the joint under investigation. Air is the additional contrast used in double contrast studies. Most often used in investigations of the knee joint but shoulder, hip, elbow and temporomandibular joints may also be imaged using this technique. The procedure is performed under strict aseptic conditions. Following the aspiration of any joint effusion the contrast agent(s) are injected into the joint. The joint is then manipulated to distribute the contrast material evenly. A mixture of fluoroscopic spot images and conventional radiographs of the region under investigation are generally acquired.

Contraindications include infection of the joint or overlying skin, and sensitivity to contrast media. Complications include joint discomfort, allergic reactions, chemical synovitis, pain, infection or capsular rupture.

NB: General anaesthesia may be required for investigation of the hip in children.

Additional modality

- Magnetic resonance imaging (MRI) has reduced the need for many of the arthrograms previously carried out in radiology departments.

Atlanto-occipital articulation
(see *also* Cervical vertebrae)

This projection demonstrates the atlanto-occipital joints visualised through the maxillary sinuses.

Basic projection

PA

- Patient prone/erect.
- Forehead and nose resting on the grid device.
- MSP perpendicular to midline of IR.
- Orbitomeatal line at 90° to IR.
- Centre to the MSP with the central ray exiting at the infraorbital margins.

Autotomography

This describes the use of patient movement, as opposed to IR and tube movement in normal tomography, to blur areas not required on the image. The most common use currently is for imaging the lateral thoracic vertebrae. The standard projection is used but the exposure is altered to include a long exposure time, e.g. 1 second. The patient continues shallow breathing during the exposure in order to blur the ribs and obtain better detail of the vertebrae and joint spaces.

Barium enema (double contrast)

Single contrast procedures, although useful in some cases, do not provide a good demonstration of the mucosal pattern. A double contrast barium enema examination generally employs the use of both fluoroscopic and conventional radiographic techniques.

Patient preparation

Prior to the examination rigorous patient preparation is essential to rid the entire large intestine of all faecal matter as this can mimic the appearance of pathology, e.g. small tumours. Patient preparation is department dependent but in general consists of the patient having a low-residue diet for 2–3 days prior to the examination with fluids only on the day before the examination. A laxative is taken the morning and evening of the day before the examination. If a bowel cleansing enema is required, it can be carried out on the day of the examination, making sure enough time is left before commencing the procedure to allow the colon to absorb the excess water this produces. Preparation is modified in patients with a predisposing condition which may be exacerbated by the usual departmental regime. In order to get the best diagnostic information from what can be a demanding examination, it is necessary to give the patient a full and comprehensive explanation of the procedure.

Technique

- Unless there is a suspicion that bowel preparation is inadequate or toxic megacolon is suspected, a control image of the abdomen is not necessary.
- A lubricated enema tube is introduced into the rectum.
- An intravenous injection of a muscle relaxant is given which will reduce bowel

peristalsis for the duration of the examination.

- The barium suspension is introduced under fluoroscopic control until it reaches the hepatic flexure.
- Spot radiographs of the bowel are taken as per department protocol and where indicated throughout the procedure.
- The barium suspension within the sigmoid colon is allowed to drain out.
- Air is gently pumped into the bowel to push the barium towards the caecum, dilate the colon and produce the double contrast effect. Patient position is manipulated to allow the barium suspension to coat the bowel mucosa.

Basic projections

Spot films under fluoroscopic control with patient lying down

- Right anterior oblique (RAO), prone and left posterior oblique (LPO) coned to the area within the rectum and sigmoid colon.
- Left lateral of the rectum.
- Left anterior oblique (LAO) with the patient tilted slightly head down to demonstrate the caecum.

Spot films under fluoroscopic control with patient erect
- LAO coned to demonstrate the splenic flexure.
- RAO coned to demonstrate the hepatic flexure.
- Coned right lateral to demonstrate the rectum.

Overcouch projections
- AP or PA left lateral decubitus to demonstrate the entire large intestine.
- AP or PA right lateral decubitus to demonstrate the entire large intestine.
- Prone abdomen with a 40° caudal angle to separate the loops of the sigmoid colon.
- Post evacuation projection of the abdomen.

Patient aftercare

The patient should be monitored until any side effects produced by the muscle relaxant have subsided. The patient should be warned that their bowel motions will be white for a few days. As residual barium suspension can cause constipation, the patient should be advised to increase their water intake.

Barium meal and follow through

A double contrast approach is preferred as this increases visualisation of the mucosal pattern. A barium sulphate suspension and a gas-producing agent provide the double contrast effect.

Patient preparation

Nil by mouth for at least 8 hours prior to the examination. It is advisable that the patient does not smoke or chew gum after midnight on the evening before the examination as both these activities increase gastric motility which is detrimental to the procedure.

Technique

- Spot films of the oesophagus are taken as the patient swallows a small amount of barium suspension under fluoroscopic control.
- The patient swallows a gas-producing agent and is advised to try not to allow the resultant gas to be ejected from their stomach.
- The barium sulphate suspension is then ingested with the patient lying on their left

side. This will increase the time it takes for the barium to reach the duodenum and to ensure that the greater curve of the stomach is not obscured.

- A muscle relaxant is then administered intravenously to aid visualisation of the gastrointestinal tract.
- The patient is manipulated by quickly turning in a complete circle to adequately coat the mucosa of the stomach.

Basic projections

Spot films under fluoroscopic control with patient lying down

- RAO, to demonstrate the antrum and greater curve of the stomach.
- Supine, to demonstrate the antrum and body of the stomach.
- LAO, to demonstrate the lesser curve of the stomach.
- Left lateral with the table tilted head up approximately 45° to demonstrate the fundus of the stomach.
- The patient then turns from a left lateral through supine, onto their left side and finally into the prone position, thus

preventing the barium suspension flowing
into the duodenal loop.
- A prone projection demonstrates the
duodenal loop.
- Four coned projections with the patient in
the prone, RAO, supine and LAO positions
demonstrate the duodenal cap.

Spot films under fluoroscopic control with
patient erect
- Projections of the fundus of the stomach.

Patient aftercare
- As for barium enema.

Barium studies

Once the exclusive domain of radiologists,
barium examinations of the gastrointestinal
tract are now increasingly the remit of
radiographers who have completed the
appropriate postgraduate courses of study.
All measures should be taken to keep the
radiation dose to both patient and practitioner
to a minimum. See Section 3 for the
contraindications to the use of barium
sulphate as the contrast medium of choice.

Muscle relaxants and gas-producing agents can also produce side effects and have contraindications that should be considered before they are administered.

Barium swallow

Patient preparation

Not necessary unless the stomach is to be examined when patient preparation is as for a barium meal.

Technique

- In the erect RAO position the patient is given a mouthful of barium suspension and asked not to swallow it.
- On command to swallow, spot films of the entire length of the oesophagus are obtained under fluoroscopic control.
- A rapid series of projections or video recording may be carried out if assessment of the laryngopharynx or the upper oesophagus is required.

Patient aftercare

Although a small quantity of barium sulphate suspension is used, the patient should still be warned that their bowel motions may be white for a few days following the examination.

Bicipital groove (see *also* Humerus; Shoulder)

To demonstrate the sulcus between the greater and lesser tuberosities on the anterior aspect of the humoral head, wherein lies the biceps tendon.

Basic projection

Inferosuperior (supine)

- Patient supine with affected arm slightly abducted and internally rotated until the sulcus is positioned anteriorly. The humeral epicondyles will be approximately 45° to the MSP.
- Patient's head rotated away from the affected side.
- IR is supported vertically on the table and in contact with the superior aspect of the shoulder.
- From the horizontal, angle the tube 5° caudally.

- Centre to the anterior humeral head.
- Exposure on arrested respiration.

Alternative projection

Inferosuperior (erect)
- Patient seated with back towards and
  30 cm away from the IR in a vertical
  stand.
- Patient leans back 30° to be in contact
  with IR.
- Affected arm abducted 30° and
  internally rotated until the sulcus is
  positioned anteriorly. The humeral
  epicondyles will be approximately 45° to
  the MSP.
- Patient's head rotated away from the
  affected side.
- From the horizontal, angle the tube 15–20°
  cranially.
- Centre to the anterior humeral head.
- Exposure on arrested respiration.

NB: The superoinferior projection is no longer
recommended as the patient dose to
radiosensitive tissues cannot be adequately
controlled.

Biliary tract

Although ultrasound is now the modality of choice, the following radiographic examinations are still performed. Contrast media can be introduced into the biliary tract orally, intravenously or by direct injection into the ducts. Each examination is named according to the route of entry and the portion of the biliary tract examined.

Basic projection

Prone LAO

- Patient prone with the left arm by the side of the body and the right arm on the pillow.
- Right hip and knee flexed slightly to raise the right side of the body (the degree of obliquity required is dependent upon patient habitus).
- Centre midway between the spine and the lateral border of the right abdominal wall at the level of the lower costal margin.
- Exposure on expiration.

NB: As only a small percentage of gallstones are visualised on plain films, this projection is now mainly used as a control prior to contrast studies.

Additional imaging

To demonstrate gall bladder function (currently rarely used).

Oral cholecystography

- The control film is taken the day before the examination, and a morning appointment arranged.
- The patient is advised to eat a light evening meal, containing no fats, prior to the examination.
- The preparatory contrast medium is taken 12 hours before the examination is due.
- No further food should be consumed although water may be taken up to 8 hours before the examination.
- A second dose of contrast may be given prior to the examination.
- Erect and prone LAO projections of the gall bladder region are acquired.
- If the gall bladder is visualised on these images, a proprietary fatty meal is given to the patient.
- A coned image in the prone LAO position is taken after 30 minutes to assess gall bladder contraction.
- In the event of the gall bladder not being demonstrated, a further examination can be

carried out on the following day after a
second dose of contrast.

Additional imaging

To demonstrate the patency of the common
bile duct and confirm/deny the presence of
any retained calculi prior to removal of the
gall bladder. This examination is carried out
during surgery.

Operative cholangiogram

- Can be carried out using traditional imaging
  methods but increasingly an image
  intensifier is used.
- Approximately 20 ml of a high-osmolar or
  low-osmolar (150 mg/ml) contrast medium
  is used.
- A LAO image of the right upper quadrant
  is taken after approximately 5 ml of
  contrast medium is injected directly into
  the common bile duct to demonstrate the
  common hepatic duct and the common
  bile duct.
- A further image after the injection of the
  remaining 15 ml of contrast should
  demonstrate the common hepatic duct, the
  common bile duct and the contrast medium
  flowing freely into the duodenum.

- The anaesthetist will arrest the patient's respiration whilst the imaging procedures take place.

Additional imaging

To assess biliary leakage or exclude retained calculi where an operative cholangiogram was not performed. A T-tube is inserted into the common bile duct in theatre, permitting healing whilst maintaining patency.

T-tube cholangiogram

- Carried out 10–14 days postoperatively.
- 20–30 ml of a high-osmolar or low-osmolar (150 mg/ml) contrast medium is used.
- A preliminary coned left anterior oblique image of the right upper quadrant is carried out.
- Contrast medium is introduced into the T-tube under fluoroscopic control and appropriate spot images taken.

Additional imaging

To guide removal of calculi percutaneously where the T-tube is withdrawn before a catheter is passed along the remaining tract. The tip is placed just beyond the calculus allowing a basket to be inserted and opened beyond the calculus. This is slowly withdrawn and the stone grasped. This procedure is carried out under fluoroscopic control.

Percutaneous extraction of retained biliary calculi
- Using fluoroscopic control and with the patient supine a needle is inserted through the lateral abdominal wall into the biliary duct.
- A guide wire is passed through the needle.
- Needle is removed.
- Catheter passed over guide wire to ROI and wire removed.
- Catheter can be left in place for extended drainage or is used to attempt to remove retained calculi using a wire basket.
- A high-osmolar or low-osmolar (150 mg/ml) contrast medium is used.

Additional imaging

Imaging of the pancreatic and biliary ducts following the introduction of a contrast medium directly into the pancreatic duct. Indications for the procedure include jaundice and pancreatic disease. The patient requires sedation.

Endoscopic retrograde
cholangiopancreatography (ERCP)

- With the patient on their left side the endoscope is introduced under fluoroscopic control until the ampulla of Vater is located.
- A cannula is passed through the endoscope and the patient pronated.
- The contrast medium is introduced to determine the correct positioning of the cannula.
- On finding calculi in the bile ducts, coned images in the prone and both oblique positions are taken.
- Images taken in the Trendelenburg position will demonstrate the intrahepatic ducts.
- To demonstrate the pancreas, coned images in the prone and both oblique positions are required.
- Delayed images may show the gall bladder (if present) and common bile duct emptying.
- To demonstrate the pancreatic duct a low-osmolar (240 mg/ml) contrast medium is used.
- To demonstrate the bile ducts a low-osmolar (150 mg/ml) contrast medium is used.

Additional imaging

To confirm or exclude extrahepatic bile duct obstruction in the jaundiced patient generally prior to intervention, e.g. drainage.

Percutaneous transhepatic
cholangiogram (PTC)

- A fluoroscopic procedure under aseptic
  conditions.
- 20–60 ml of low-osmolar (150 mg/ml)
  contrast medium is used.
- A preliminary projection of the right upper
  quadrant is performed and contrast injected
  until the full ductal system is demonstrated.
- Post-injection projections that may be
  required include 45° obliques, right lateral,
  projections in the Trendelenburg position,
  spot projections of the gall bladder and
  delayed images to show contrast in the gall
  bladder.

Additional modalities

- US is the modality of choice as it
  demonstrates good visualisation of the
  liver parenchyma, gall bladder and ducts,
  although the pancreas is not always well
  demonstrated. It is non-invasive, generally
  readily available and with no radiation dose
  to the patient. Indications include pain,
  jaundice, acute pancreatitis and assessment
  of gall bladder function or gallstones. The
  only preparation required is the need for a
  patient to fast. Ultrasound can also be used
  to guide percutaneous procedures.

- CT provides good visualisation of the pancreas, liver, gall bladder and ducts.
- MRI in the form of magnetic resonance cholangiopancreatography (MRCP) provides excellent visualisation of the biliary tract, pancreatic duct and gall bladder without contrast media administration, instrumentation or radiation and therefore entails less risk than ERCP.
- RNI for acute cholecystitis can identify an obstructed gall bladder from a hepatobiliary iminodiacetic acid (HIDA) scan. Biliary scintigraphy can also be of use in chronic cholecystitis.

Bitewing radiography

To demonstrate the crowns of the upper and lower premolar and molar teeth in occlusion, on one IR. The long axis of the IR can be placed horizontally or vertically as per clinical indications. The interdental spaces should be well demonstrated if the IR is parallel to the teeth and the CR perpendicular to both.

Basic projections

It is recommended that IR holders and a beam aiming device are used to aid accurate patient positioning and the correct alignment of the x-ray tube head. This will help to ensure optimum image quality and avoid the common fault of cone cutting. A bitewing acquired using the traditional detachable tab is operator dependent and not generally reproducible.

Molar region
- Position appropriately sized IR with its anterior edge opposite the distal aspect of the lower canine.
- Close patient's mouth slowly until the teeth are in occlusion.
- Ensure occlusal plane is parallel to the horizontal axis of the IR.
- Using the beam aiming device, the CR is directed through the contacts of the teeth.

Premolar region
- Positioning as above with appropriate alteration to the position of the x-ray tubehead.
- Using the beam aiming device, the CR is directed through the contacts of the teeth.

Bladder (*see also* Cystography; Cystourethrography; Intravenous urography)

Basic projection

AP

- Patient supine with no rotation of the pelvis.
- 15° caudal angulation to the MSP.
- Centre 5 cm above the upper border of the symphysis pubis.

Additional modality

- US is now more often the modality of choice for bladder investigation in the first instance.

Bone age (*see* Wrist)

To establish the skeletal age of a child with retarded development of stature for chronological age, e.g. in Perthes' disease. The PA projection of the left wrist is usually taken for comparison with images from the Greulich and Pyle[1] Atlas or for use with the Tanner and Whitehouse[2] scoring system.

Breast (see Mammography)

Bronchi (see Chest; Foreign bodies)

Calcaneum (see *also* Ankle; Foot)

Basic projections 18×24cm   Fine Focus

To demonstrate a fracture. 100cm FFD

Lateral
* Patient positioned as for the lateral ankle.
* Centre 2.5 cm below and 2.5 cm behind the medial malleolus.

Axial
* Patient positioned as for the AP ankle.
* Tube angled 60° cranially.
* Centre to the midline of the plantar aspect of the heel, 1 cm below the base of the 5th metatarsal.
* A bandage may be placed around the forefoot and held by the patient in order to maintain dorsiflexion.
* Both calcanei can be imaged on one exposure by centring between the heels.

Additional projection

To demonstrate calcaneal spur and Severs' disease (osteochondritis).

Lateral
• Projection of affected calcaneum.

NB: These patients can often be managed without imaging.

Carpal tunnel (see *also* Wrist)

Basic projection

To demonstrate bony causes of pressure on the nerves of the hand as they pass through the carpal tunnel.

Tangential/inferosuperior
• Patient seated with the forearm parallel to the long axis of the table.
• Hyperextend wrist and position the long axis of hand as near vertical as possible.
• Ask patient to hold hand and thumb in this position with the unaffected hand and a bandage to avoid unnecessary exposure.

- Tube angled 25–30° cranially.
- Centre 2.5 cm distal to the base of the 3rd metacarpal.

Alternative projection

This position is often easier for the patient to maintain.

Superoinferior
- The patient stands with their back to the examination table.
- Dorsiflex the wrist.
- Move the patient's arm posteriorly to place the hand and wrist over the IR, forearm as near vertical as possible.
- Angle the tube 20–35° cranially to enter the midpoint of the wrist.

Cephalometry

Used in orthodontic assessment to ensure standardisation of patient position and allow comparisons to be made throughout a course of treatment. The procedure allows specific measurements to be made within the facial skeleton.

SECTION
2

Basic projection

Lateral

- Patient erect, either standing or sitting.
- MSP parallel to the IR and Frankfort plane parallel to the floor.
- CR perpendicular to MSP and the IR to enter through the external auditory meatuses (EAM).
- Patient's head is immobilised within the cephalostat with the ear rods gently and gradually inserted into the EAMs.
- An additional aluminium wedge filter placed between the patient and the anterior aspect of the IR allows visualisation of the soft tissue profile.

NB: The resultant image should be a true lateral projection with the ear rods superimposed on one another.

Cervical ribs (see *also* Chest)

Basic projection

To demonstrate supernumerary ribs arising from C7.

Modified AP

- Patient supine/erect with the chin elevated.
- Tube angled 10° cranially.

- Centre to the MSP, 2.5 cm above the sternal notch.

NB: Cervical ribs may also be demonstrated on PA and apical projections of the chest.

Cervical vertebrae

Plain radiological investigation of the cervical vertebrae is no longer routine for patients complaining of neck pain or for investigation of myelopathy, MRI being the modality of choice. Cervical vertebrae projections are indicated for trauma cases involving neck injury with pain or neurological deficit, or for any unconscious patient with head injury. In this event careful patient management is required. Never remove an immobilising device and ensure there is as little movement of the patient as possible until the extent of the injury is established. Any movement should be supervised by the referring medical practitioner. The initial radiograph should be a lateral projection obtained using a horizontal beam, and assessed before moving on to the AP C3–C7. Imaging C7/T1 in the

lateral position may require assistance from
the referring medical practitioner with pulling
the shoulders down and away from the area
of interest. An additional projection (*see*
Cervicothoracic junction) may be required.

Basic projections

24 x 30cm [handwritten]

Lateral C1–C7 *180cm Fine Focus* [handwritten]

- Patient sitting/standing erect with the
  shoulder of the affected side in contact with
  the lower border of the IR in a true lateral
  position, chin slightly raised.
- Shoulders relaxed and arms placed slightly
  behind the back.
- Centre 2.5 cm behind and 5 cm below the
  angle of the mandible over C3. *THYROID EMINENCE* [handwritten]
- The SID for this projection is 180 cm.

AP C3–C7 *100cm Broad Focus 18x24cm* [handwritten]

- Patient erect/supine with the MSP
  perpendicular to the IR.
- Raise chin to superimpose the lower border
  of the mandible over the occiput.
- With a horizontal or vertical central ray,
  angle the tube 15° cephalad.
- Centre to the MSP to enter the patient at the
  level of C4.

Additional projections

AP C1–C2 100cm Fine focus 18×24cm

- Patient erect/supine in the true AP position with chin slightly raised.

- Upper occlusal plane perpendicular to the IR, i.e. radiographic baseline at approximately 10° to the IR.
- Centre to the MSP, 2.5 cm below upper lip.
- Before exposure the patient must open the mouth as wide as possible without moving from this position.

Flexion and extension projections can detect ligamentous injury and aid preoperative planning for arthritic patients requiring general anaesthetic. Both projections are performed.

Lateral projections in flexion/extension
- Patient positioned as for the lateral projection.
- Image taken in full flexion of the neck (patient drops head forwards and draws chin as close to chest as possible).
- Image taken with the neck fully extended (patient elevates chin as much as possible).
- Centre as for lateral C1–C7.

NB: Images should be labelled appropriately.

Oblique projections will demonstrate subluxation and narrowing of the intervertebral foramina.

Posterior oblique C1–C7

- From the lateral position the patient is rotated back 45°.
- The head is turned so that the MSP is parallel to the IR and the chin is raised.
- Tube angled 15° cranially.
- Centre to the angle of the mandible furthest from the IR.
- SID of 180 cm is used.
- Both obliques may be required for comparison.

NB: This projection demonstrates the intervertebral foramina of the side furthest away from the IR.

Alternative projections

AP oblique projections may be performed but deliver an increased dose to the thyroid.

Anterior oblique C1–C7

- From the lateral position the patient is rotated 45° towards the IR.
- The head is turned so that the MSP is parallel to the IR and the chin is raised.

- Tube angled 15° cranially.
- Centre to the midline of the cervical vertebrae at the level of the angle of the mandible.
- SID of 180 cm is used.
- Both obliques may be required for comparison.

NB: These projections demonstrate the intervertebral foramina of the side nearest the IR.

Additional modalities

- The higher contrast resolution of CT provides improved visualisation of a subtle fracture. It can classify fractures and identify any compromise of the vertebral canal. It can, however, be difficult to identify fractures in the axial plane and is unable to show ligamentous injuries.
- MRI demonstrates excellent soft tissue contrast and provides diagnostic information in different planes. It has the ability to demonstrate the vertebral arteries. Importantly no ionising radiation is used. However, there is loss of bony detail on the resultant images.

Cervicothoracic Junction (see also Cervical vertebrae)

To demonstrate the cervicothoracic region in patients whose body habitus prevents visualisation of C7 and T1 on the basic lateral cervical projection.

Cervicothoracic (Swimmer's)
- Patient positioned as for the lateral projection, either supine or erect with shoulder nearer the tube depressed.
- Arm nearer the IR raised above the head.
- Centre 1 cm above the shoulder nearer the tube.
- The normal lateral exposure should be increased by approximately 7 kVp to penetrate the shoulder region sufficiently.

NB: This projection will demonstrate C7 and T1 projected between the shoulders.

Chest

To demonstrate pulmonary pathology and the cardiac outline. Routinely indicated if the patient has acute or central chest pain, haemoptysis, suspected pleural effusion, inhaled

foreign body, as a follow-up to pneumonia or
cardiac disease, for cancer staging and for
patients in ITU/HDU (although the value of a
daily chest x-ray for the latter is in question).

Basic projection FINE FOCUS
PA ~~Program~~ 180cm   35 X 43cm

- Patient in the erect position with the
  anterior chest against the IR, chin raised
  and supported on top of the IR.
- Backs of the hands placed on the hips, elbows
  rotated forwards and shoulders relaxed.
- Centre in the midline to the level of T6/T7.
- Exposure on full inspiration.
- SID for this projection is 180 cm.

NB: If an air-gap technique is used, the SID is
usually increased to 360 cm (a minimum of
300 cm is required).

Alternative projections

If the patient cannot assume the position
described above.

AP
- Patient in the erect position with the
  posterior aspect of the chest against the IR
  and the chin raised slightly.

- Shoulders relaxed and arms internally rotated.
- Centre in the midline to the level of T6/T7.
- Exposure on full inspiration.
- SID for this projection is 180 cm.

NB: This projection does not always clear the scapulae from the lung fields and magnifies the heart, preventing accurate measurement of the cardiothoracic ratio.

Lateral decubitus (PA) *fine focus 180cm No grid 35×43cm*

To demonstrate fluid the patient lies on their affected side. To demonstrate air in the pleural cavity the patient lies on their unaffected side.

- Knees flexed and arms raised above head.
- IR placed in vertical holder with long axis parallel to table top.
- Anterior aspect of chest in contact with IR, ensuring that all of thorax is included.
- Centre to MSP at T7.
- Exposure on full inspiration.

NB: Allow patient to remain in this position for at least 5 minutes before exposure.

Lateral decubitus (AP)

If patient condition will not allow a PA projection an AP can be performed.

- Knees flexed and arms raised above head.
- IR placed in vertical holder with long axis parallel to table top.
- Posterior aspect of chest in contact with IR, ensuring that all of thorax is included.
- Centre to MSP at T7.
- Exposure on full inspiration.

Additional projection

The lateral projection is required only if pathology is indicated. A left lateral projection is taken by default if there is no affected side unless the projection is taken for evaluation of the lung volume in cystic fibrosis, when a right lateral projection is performed.

Lateral
- Patient in the erect position with the side under examination against the IR.
- Hands placed on the head with elbows together (or arms supported clear of the chest).
- Centre at the mid-coronal plane at the level of the axilla (T6).
- SID for this projection is 180 cm.

Additional projection

To demonstrate lesions in the apices (e.g. metastatic disease, tuberculosis) by projecting the clavicles above the apices of the lungs.

Apical (horizontal beam)
- Patient sitting/standing facing the tube, 30 cm in front of the IR.
- Recline the trunk until the shoulders are in contact with the IR and the angle of the coronal plane is 30° to the IR.
- Arms and hands internally rotated.
- Centre to the MSP at the level of the sternal angle (T4).
- Exposure on full inspiration.
- SID for this projection is 180 cm.

Alternative projection

If the patient cannot assume the position described above.

Apical (angled beam)
- Patient sitting/standing facing the tube, back in contact with the IR.
- Arms and hands internally rotated.
- Tube angled 30° cranially.
- Centre to the MSP at the level of the sternal angle (T4).
- Exposure on full inspiration.
- SID for this projection is 180 cm.

Additional projection

To demonstrate right middle lobe collapse or interlobular pleural effusion.

Lordotic
- Patient erect facing the IR.
- Grasping the sides of the vertical bucky for support, the patient leans backwards through 30–45°.
- Centre to the MSP at the level of the axilla (T6).
- Exposure on full inspiration.
- SID for this projection is 180 cm.

Additional projections

To demonstrate the aorta separated from the heart and vertebral column.

RAO
- Patient erect facing the IR with right shoulder in contact.
- Right hand on the right hip and left hand on the head.
- Rotate the left side of the body 60° away from the IR.
- Centre to the medial border of the scapula further away from the IR at the level of T5/T6.
- Exposure on full inspiration.
- SID for this projection is 180 cm.

LAO

- Patient erect facing the IR with left shoulder in contact.
- Left hand on the left hip and right hand on the head.
- Rotate the right side of the body 70° away from the IR.
- Centre to the medial border of the scapula further away from the IR at the level of T5/T6.
- Exposure on full inspiration.
- SID for this projection is 180 cm.

Additional projection

To demonstrate or exclude a pneumothorax following penetrating/moderate chest trauma, or in patients with suspected inhalation of a foreign body.

PA (in expiration)

- Patient in the erect position with the anterior chest against the IR and the chin raised.
- Backs of the hands placed on the hips, elbows rotated forwards and shoulders relaxed.
- Centre in the midline to the level of the axilla (T6).
- Exposure on full expiration.
- SID for this projection is 180 cm.

Additional modalities

- Transthoracic or transoesophageal ultrasound can detect aortic dissection and provide dynamic imaging of the chambers and valves of the heart.
- CT can be used to exclude other causes of acute chest pain in conjunction with US.
- MRI is increasingly used to identify suspected aortic dissection and monitor progress.
- RNI provides perfusion information in patients with suspected myocardial infarction.

Cholangiography (see Biliary tract)

Clavicle

Basic projections

To demonstrate a fracture of the clavicle (usually occurs in the middle third).

PA 100cm FINE Focus 24×30cm

- Patient erect/prone.
- Rotate unaffected side away from IR 10–15° until clavicle of affected side is in close contact with the IR.

- Patient's head rotated away from the affected side.
- Centre to the middle of the clavicle.
- Exposure on arrested respiration.

Inferosuperior
- Patient erect facing the tube with the affected clavicle parallel to the IR.
- Patient leans back by approximately 30°.
- Patient's head rotated away from the affected side.
- Tube angled 20° cranially.
- Centre to the middle of the clavicle.
- Exposure on arrested respiration.

NB: This projection projects the clavicle clear of the chest wall and demonstrates displacement of fragments in the event of a fracture.

Alternative projection

If the PA position is impossible for the patient to attain due to injury.

AP
- Patient erect/supine.
- Rotate body 10–15° until clavicle of affected side is parallel to the IR.
- Patient's head rotated away from the affected side.

- Centre to the middle of the clavicle.
- Exposure on arrested respiration.

Coccyx

To demonstrate pathology, but mainly fracture or subluxation of the coccyx. Faecal matter can be problematic when imaging the coccyx and the bladder should be empty to improve visualisation of the ROI.

Basic projections

AP
- Patient supine with hips and knees flexed.
- Tube angled 10–15° caudally dependent on patient habitus.
- Centre to the MSP, 2.5 cm above the symphysis pubis.

Lateral
- Patient lying in the true lateral position.
- Centre 9 cm posterior and 5 cm inferior to the anterior superior iliac spine (ASIS).

NB: Radiation protection for female patients cannot be used on these projections and, therefore, the request should be carefully considered if the patient is of childbearing age.

Coracoid process (see Shoulder)

Cranium (see Skull)

Cystography (see *also* Cystourethrography)

Cystography is a retrograde procedure with
the preferred choice of contrast medium
being non-ionic and with a lower
concentration than that used for intravenous
urogram (IVU) examinations due to the large
volume of contrast required to fill the bladder.
The procedure can be performed in theatre or
the radiology department. The patient may
arrive with a catheter in situ in the bladder.
If not, catheterisation will take place in the
x-ray department under strict aseptic
conditions. Prior to insertion of the catheter
the patient will be required to empty their
bladder. With the patient supine a preliminary
radiograph of the bladder region is performed
(*see* Bladder). A catheter is then introduced
into the bladder via the urethral canal, any
residual urine drained and the contrast
medium introduced under fluoroscopic
control.

Basic projections

AP bladder
- As for routine bladder.

NB: Ureteric reflux may be demonstrated with the patient straining.

Obliques
- From the AP position, rotate the patient 50–60° to either side in turn.
- Tube angled 10° caudally.
- Direct the CR to enter the patient 5 cm above the upper border of the symphysis pubis and 5 cm medial to the ASIS of the raised side.
- Exposure on suspended respiration.

Cystourethrography

This procedure has been used to investigate such conditions as vesicoureteric reflux, abnormalities of the urethra and bladder, abnormal external genitalia in children and stress incontinence. However, the radiation dose involved in a micturating cystourethrogram should preclude it being used as a first-line investigation.

To demonstrate the urethra and neck of the bladder in the male, the bladder is emptied prior to the examination and a preliminary image of the area is obtained. With the patient supine and in the oblique position, a urethral syringe containing the required amount of contrast medium is attached to a device sited in the urethral orifice. The contrast medium is slowly administered under fluoroscopic control so that transitory reflux is not missed. Projections in the AP and oblique positions are taken as required as the contrast fills the urethra. Post examination, a full length image or fluoroscopic projections of the kidneys may be obtained to identify any refluxed contrast medium.

Additional modality

- RNI has largely replaced the micturating cystourethrogram.

Dacrocystography

The radiographic investigation of the lacrimal system following injection of a contrast medium. Macroradiography is sometimes employed for this procedure to aid demonstration of the site and assess the degree of obstruction of the lacrimal passages (obstructive epiphora). Under aseptic conditions, local anaesthesia, if required, is applied to the conjunctiva. The lower lacrimal punctum is dilated and a fine cannula or nylon catheter inserted. This is attached to a syringe containing a warmed, oil-based contrast medium which is then injected into the duct. Images are obtained prior to and immediately after introduction of the contrast medium. Delayed images may be required.

Basic projections

Modified occipitomental
- Patient erect/prone.
- Radiographic baseline at 35° to horizontal.
- Centre at the lower orbital margin of the affected side.

Lateral
- Patient erect/supine.
- Affected side towards the IR.
- Centre to the lower orbital margin.

Dental panoramic tomography (DPT)
(see Orthopantomography)

An extraoral technique used to examine the mandible, maxilla, temporomandibular joints and the teeth on a single image. The specialised DPT machine allows the imaging of one layer or section, in the shape of the dental arches, while blurring images from structures in other planes. This is achieved by the tube and IR moving horizontally around the patient's head. It is a relatively simple technique which allows rapid assessment with a reduction in the radiation dose that would have been received had individual periapicals been performed.

The patient is erect and positioned in the machine with the Frankfort plane horizontal and the MSP perpendicular to the floor. The patient is instructed to place the groove in the bite peg between their front teeth, the chin positioned on the chin support and the shoulders relaxed.

Holding the support handles the patient steps slightly forward into the machine to ensure that the cervical spine is vertical. The head clamps are applied to immobilise the patient. Prior to exposure the patient is requested to close their lips and press their tongue to the roof of their mouth.

A major disadvantage of the long exposure times required for this procedure can be patient movement. This problem may be reduced by demonstration of tube movement prior to patient positioning. Another disadvantage of this technique is that the fine detail of the individual teeth is not optimal. Precise patient positioning is important to reduce the likelihood of a reduction in the quality of the resultant image. Some common positioning errors are mentioned here.

- Chin too high or too low results in distortion in the shape of the mandible with the anterior teeth out of focus.
- Head too far forward results in narrowed, blurred incisors.
- Head too far back results in widened, blurred incisors.
- Lips open results in dark radiolucent shadow obscuring anterior teeth.
- Tongue not to roof of mouth results in dark radiolucent shadow obscuring apices of maxillary teeth.
- Mid-sagittal plane incorrect results in ramus and posterior teeth appearing magnified. Side closer to the IR also appears smaller.
- Spine position incorrect results in the cervical spine appearing as a radiopacity in the centre of the film, obscuring diagnostic information.

NB: Owing to the length of the exposure, panoramic tomography is not considered to be suitable for very young children.

Dental radiography (see Bitewing radiography; Cephalometry; Dental panoramic tomography; Occlusal radiography; Periapical radiography)

Diaphragm

To demonstrate formation of a subphrenic abscess or perforation in the abdominal cavity. Plain radiographic techniques, e.g. erect chest, erect abdomen including the diaphragm, lateral or dorsal decubitus projections of the region, will demonstrate any free gas collecting under the diaphragm. Paralysis of the diaphragm, and certain pathologies above or below the diaphragm, can also affect its normal position and movement. These are usually examined under fluoroscopic control during breathing exercises. An alternative radiological examination of the diaphragm involves two separate exposures on one IR, one in full inspiration and one in full expiration, using half the usual exposure for each. Care should be taken to prevent patient movement between exposures.

Discography

Additional modalities

- CT is used to diagnose disc herniations and protrusions. It is the preferred modality when a patient presents with sciatic pain and can be used with contrast media to improve the detection of pathology.
- MRI is of equal or increased sensitivity in the diagnosis of disc disorders.

Elbow (see *also* Olecranon process; Radial head; Ulnar groove)

Basic projections

To demonstrate bony injury or pathology.

AP 24 x 30cm Fine focus 100cm

- Patient sitting with affected side parallel to examination table.
- Upper extremity in the same horizontal plane as IR.
- Fully extend elbow joint and supinate hand, rotating from shoulder joint only.
- Humeral epicondyles equidistant from IR.
- Centre 2.5 cm distal to the midpoint between the humeral epicondyles.

Lateral 24 × 30 cm FINE FOCUS 100cm

- From the AP position, internally rotate upper extremity 90°.
- Elbow flexed 90°, humeral epicondyles superimposed.
- Centre to the lateral epicondyle of the humerus.

Alternative projections

In cases where the patient is unable to extend the elbow, the following techniques may be employed to obtain the most diagnostic images of the areas of interest in the elbow joint.

To demonstrate the distal humerus.

AP in partial flexion
- The humerus should be in the same horizontal plane as the shoulder and in contact with the IR.
- Extend the elbow as far as the patient finds comfortable and support the forearm.
- Supinate the hand if possible.
- Centre midway between the humeral epicondyles.

NB: The proximal radius and ulna will be distorted on this projection.

To demonstrate the proximal radius and ulna.

AP in partial flexion
- With the elbow extended as far as is comfortable, the patient is positioned with the dorsal surface of the forearm in contact with the IR.
- Supinate the hand if possible.
- Centre to a point 2.5 cm below the humeral epicondyles in the midline.

NB: The distal humerus will appear distorted in this projection.

To demonstrate the elbow joint.

AP in partial flexion
- With the point of the elbow in contact with the IR, the patient is adjusted so that the angles between the humerus and the table top and the forearm and the table top are equidistant.
- Support the humerus and the forearm.
- Supinate the hand if possible.
- Centre to the crease of the elbow joint in the midline.

NB: This projection demonstrates the entire joint with equal amounts of distortion to the distal humerus and the proximal radius and ulna.

Alternative projections

For the patient who presents with their arm in acute flexion the following techniques may be employed to obtain the most diagnostic AP images of the areas of interest in the elbow joint.

To demonstrate the distal humerus.

AP in acute flexion
- The elbow and shoulder joints should be in the same horizontal plane.
- Place the fully flexed elbow onto the IR and ensure that there is no rotation of the limb.
- Centre 5 cm superior to the olecranon process.

NB: The distal humerus and proximal radius and ulna are superimposed but the olecranon process should be clearly demonstrated.

To demonstrate the proximal radius and ulna.

AP in acute flexion
- The elbow and shoulder joints should be in the same horizontal plane.
- Place the fully flexed elbow onto the IR which is displaced towards the shoulder and ensure that there is no rotation of the limb.
- Angle the tube cranially to a degree that is perpendicular to the forearm.
- Centre 5 cm superior to the olecranon process.

NB: The distal humerus and proximal radius and ulna are superimposed. This projection provides better visualisation of the elbow joint than the projection used to demonstrate the distal humerus.

Alternative projection

For the patient who presents with limited elbow or shoulder movement or has an arm immobilised across their chest in a sling.

Lateral
- Patient supine or erect.
- Do not remove the arm from the sling.
- Place lead protection across the patient's trunk.
- Slide the IR between the medial aspect of the elbow and the patient's body.
- Ensure stability of the IR.
- Centre a horizontal beam to the lateral epicondyle of the humerus.
- Exposure on arrested respiration.

Additional projections

In paediatric patients, views of both elbows are sometimes requested for comparison of ossification centres, but these should no longer be carried out as routine.

Endoscopic retrograde cholangiopancreatography (ERCP) (see Biliary tract)

Extraoral dental radiography (see Cephalometry; Dental panoramic tomography; Sialography (Lateral oblique mandible))

Eye

To demonstrate the presence of radiopaque foreign bodies (FBs) in the eye or orbital cavity. If a film/screen combination is used, the screens should be cleaned immediately prior to the examination to avoid artefacts confusing the diagnosis.

Basic projections

Occipitomental (OM)
- Patient erect/prone with nose and chin resting on grid device.
- Radiographic baseline at 45° to IR.
- Centre to the MSP at the level of the lower orbital margins.
- Reduce exposure by approximately 5 kVp to demonstrate soft tissues.

NB: This projection is often used prior to an MRI investigation if the patient has worked with metallic materials or power tools. A positive finding would be a contraindication to proceeding with the MRI.

Lateral
- Patient erect/supine with head in true lateral position.
- Eyes facing straight ahead.
- Centre to the outer canthus of the eye nearest the tube.
- Reduce exposure by approximately 5 kVp to demonstrate soft tissues.

Additional projection

To better demonstrate the position of a foreign body if detected.

Lateral
- Patient erect/supine with head in true lateral position.
- Centre to the outer canthus of the eye nearest the tube.
- Reduce exposure by approximately 5 kVp to demonstrate soft tissues.
- One exposure is made with the eyes in each of the following positions:

1. looking up
2. looking down.

NB: If the FB moves up with projection (1) and down with (2), it must be positioned on the anterior aspect of the eye or muscles. Conversely, a more posterior FB will move down with projection (1) and up with (2).

Additional modalities

- CT scans are the modality of choice for metallic intraorbital foreign body localisation. However, it should be noted that they are of limited value when non-metallic foreign bodies are involved or when a metallic foreign body is close to the sclera.
- US is a useful adjunct tool in localising and determining if the object is metallic. In addition, it may aid in the detection of retinal and choroidal detachments. Development of ultrasound biomicroscopy has helped in the localisation of intraorbital foreign bodies in the anterior segment of the eye.
- MRI is not used where metallic foreign bodies are suspected but may be more effective in localising those that are non-metallic.

Facial bones

To demonstrate bony injury to the orbits, middle third and mandibular region of the face following trauma. Nasal trauma is no longer imaged routinely as the correlation between external deformity and radiological findings is not high.

Basic projections

OM
- Patient erect/prone with nose and chin resting on grid device.
- Radiographic baseline at 45° to IR.
- Centre to the MSP to emerge at the level of the lower orbital margins.

30° OM
- Patient positioned as for the OM projection.
- Tube angled 30° caudally.
- Centre to the MSP at the level of the lower orbital margins.

Lateral
- Patient erect/supine with MSP parallel to the IR.
- Centre 2.5 cm below the outer canthus of the eye nearest the tube.

Fallopian tubes (see Hysterosalpingography)

Femur

It is essential to have at least one joint demonstrated on the resultant image, i.e. nearest the region of the femur under investigation. If the whole of the shaft of an adult femur is to be imaged, two projections may be required.

Basic projections

AP *100cm   BROAD Focus   35×43cm*

- Patient supine.
- Centre the midline of the affected femur to the midline of the IR.
- Displace the IR to include the joint of choice.
- Rotate the lower limb internally to bring the neck of the femur parallel to the IR.
- Centre to the midline of the femur at the centre of the IR.

Lateral (distal femur and knee) *100cm Broad Focus*

- Patient turned to affected side with knee *35×43cm* flexed and ankle supported on a pad.
- Opposite leg removed from the ROI by placing it behind/in front of the affected limb.
- Ensure femoral condyles are superimposed.

- Centre to the midline of the femur at the centre of the IR.

Lateral oblique (proximal femur and hip)
- From the supine position rotate the patient 45° towards the affected side, and support.
- Flex affected hip, rotate knee outwards until in a true lateral position and in contact with the table top.
- Top of IR at ASIS.
- Centre to the midline of the femur at the crease of the groin.

Alternative projections

A suspected fracture of the femur will necessitate adaptations to ensure minimal patient movement.

Horizontal beam lateral (distal femur and knee)
- With the patient supine, carefully place pads under the affected hip and knee to raise the femur above the mattress.
- The vertical IR is positioned against the medial aspect of the affected femur.
- Region of interest (ROI) to include knee joint with femoral condyles superimposed.
- Support the IR in position.

- Centre a horizontal beam perpendicular to the centre of the IR.

Horizontal beam lateral (proximal femur and hip)

- With the patient supine, carefully place pads under the affected hip and knee to raise the femur above the mattress.
- Flex the knee of the unaffected limb and elevate the foot to prevent superimposition of the legs.
- Support the raised limb and ensure that there is no rotation of the pelvis.
- The vertical gridded IR is positioned at 45° to the lateral aspect of the affected femur with its upper edge pushed gently into the patient's waist. The neck of the femur should be parallel to the IR.
- Support the IR in position.
- Centre a horizontal beam perpendicular to the centre of the IR through the neck of the femur.

Fibula (see *also* Tibia)

Basic projections

The basic projections for the fibula also include the tibia.

AP 1000cm Fine Focus 35 × 43cm

- Patient supine/seated with the affected
  lower limb resting on the IR.
- Dorsiflex foot to avoid superimposition of
  the calcaneum on the tibiotalar joint space.
- Internally rotate the lower limb to bring the
  malleoli equidistant from the IR.
- Centre to the centre of the IR.

NB: The head of fibula is occluded by the tibial
plateau on this projection.

Lateral 1000cm Fine Focus 35 × 43cm

- Patient rotated to the affected side with knee
  flexed and supported on a pad.
- Lateral aspect of the lower limb resting on
  the IR with malleoli superimposed.
- Centre midway between the knee and ankle
  joints.

Additional projection

To demonstrate the head of fibula clearly.

AP with medial rotation
- Patient supine/seated with the affected
  lower limb resting on the IR.
- Dorsiflex foot to avoid superimposition of the
  calcaneum on the tibiotalar joint space.
- Rotate the entire limb 45° medially.

• Centre midway between the knee and the
ankle joints.

Fingers (see *also* Hand, Thumb)

Basic projections   *18 × 24cm*

PA (2nd to 5th)   *100cm Fine focus*

• Patient seated.
• Place the extended digit(s) palmar surface
down directly onto the IR.
• Centre the IR to the proximal
interphalangeal (PIP) joints.
• Centre to the PIP of the affected digit.   *18 × 24cm*

Lateral (2nd and 3rd)   *100cm Fine focus*

• From the PA position, medially rotate the
hand through 90° until lateral aspect of
index finger is in contact with the IR.
• Separate the digits.
• Centre the IR to the PIP joints.
• Centre to the PIP of the affected digit.

Lateral (4th and 5th)

• From the PA position, laterally rotate the
hand through 90° until medial aspect of 5th
digit is in contact with the IR.
• Separate the extended digits.
• Centre the IR to the PIP joints.
• Centre to the PIP of the affected digit.

Foot

long axis of foot with long axis of IR use 15° Pad

Basic projections *FINE FOCUS*

Dorsiplantar (DP) *24 x 30 IR*

- Patient supine/sitting with the knee of the affected side flexed.
- Sole of the affected foot resting on the IR.
- Centre to the base of the 3rd metatarsal.

DP oblique

- From the DP position, rotate the leg medially to raise the lateral aspect of the foot until an angle of 30° is formed between the plantar surface of the foot and the IR.
- Centre to the base of the third metatarsal.

Lateral

- Patient supine.
- Rotate patient towards the affected side with the knee and hip flexed.
- Plantar surface of the foot perpendicular to the IR.
- Dorsiflex the foot.
- Centre to the navicular, cuniform region.

Additional projection

To demonstrate the relationship between the joints of the tarsal bones and the metatarsals.

Lateral weight-bearing
• Patient standing with weight equally
  distributed between feet.
• Feet in true lateral position.
• IR supported against the medial aspect of
  the foot under investigation.
• Provide lead protection between IR and
  contralateral foot.
• Centre to the tubercle of the 5th metatarsal.

Foramen magnum (see Skull)

Forearm

Basic projections   NO GRID

AP 100 FFD   FINE Focus   24 × 30cm

• Patient seated with the upper extremity in
  same horizontal plane as the IR.
• Fully extend the elbow joint and supinate
  the hand, rotating from the shoulder joint.
• Humeral epicondyles equidistant from the
  IR.
• Centre to the midpoint of the forearm.

Lateral 100 FFD   FINE Focus   24 × 30cm

• Patient seated with the upper extremity in
  same horizontal plane as the IR.

- The forearm is placed with the ulnar border of the hand and forearm in contact with the IR and the elbow flexed to 90°.
- The humeral epicondyles and the radial and ulnar styloid processes should be superimposed and perpendicular to the IR.
- Centre to the midpoint of the forearm.

Foreign bodies (see *also* Eye)

The method of imaging is dependent upon the size, degree of opacity, method of introduction and location of the FB.

Percutaneous
Glass, metal or wood splinters generally require two projections at right angles to each other with a radiopaque marker placed adjacent to the site of entry. Include the skin surface and a large area around the entry site on the resultant radiograph. AP and lateral projections are the usual projections of choice; however, a tangential projection may be helpful in establishing the depth of FBs in certain cases, e.g. scalp, and may demonstrate relationships to bone. Exposure factors must demonstrate bone and soft tissue detail.

Ingested

The three most common sites for lodging of FBs are the thoracic inlet, mid-oesophagus (where the aortic arch and carina overlap the oesophagus on a chest x-ray) and the lower oesophageal sphincter (cardiac sphincter). However, the majority pass without complication into the stomach and through the small and large intestines.

In small children a single AP projection will generally demonstrate the entire alimentary tract. A lateral soft tissue of the neck and oropharynx is required if the FB is not demonstrated.

For the larger child an AP projection of the neck and chest, followed by an AP of the abdomen are carried out. Overlap of the two projections is essential. Again, soft tissue lateral projections of the neck and oropharynx may be required if the FB is not located. Follow-up images may be required.

Adults require an AP projection of the neck and chest, followed by an AP of the abdomen if the object is sharp, potentially poisonous or large enough to cause an obstruction. Overlap of the two projections is essential. A lateral projection with a suitable soft tissue exposure to demonstrate the pharynx and the upper oesophagus is also required.

Localisation by means of coating the FB with contrast medium under fluoroscopic control may aid in the detection of non-opaque FBs. Again, follow-up radiographs may be required.

Inhaled

Inhaled FBs can result in minimal symptoms or lead to respiratory compromise, failure and even death. Common FBs inhaled by children are teeth and peanuts whilst adults present most commonly with vegetable matter, meat, bones or dental appliances. They may lodge in the larynx, trachea or right main bronchus. Small objects may occlude smaller bronchial branches. As a result collapse to part of the lung may be demonstrated even if the FB is radiolucent. A PA projection of the chest in full inspiration is required. An additional PA projection exposed on full expiration may also be required.

Intraocular
See Eye.

Additional modalities

- CT, with its greater contrast resolution, can sometimes demonstrate FBs in the airway that are radiolucent on plain radiographs. CT is also useful for gauging the relationship of the FB to organs.

- MRI can be used for non-metallic FBs, e.g. inhaled peanuts have a high fat content which gives a high-intensity signal surrounded by the low intensity of the lung fields.
- Nuclear medicine in the form of a perfusion lung scan will demonstrate areas of decreased ventilation.
- US is extremely useful for identifying FBs near radiosensitive areas.

Glenohumeral joint (see Shoulder)

Hallux valgus (see Toes)

Hand

Basic projections

NO GRID

PA 100FFD FINE FOCUS 24 × 30cm

- Patient seated with elbow flexed.
- Place hand, palmar surface down, onto IR.
- Fingers and thumb slightly separated and fully extended.
- Centre to the head of the 3rd metacarpal.

PA oblique IOOFD *No Grid Fine focus*

- From the PA position rotate the hand 45° towards the lateral border.
- Slightly flex and separate the fingers and support on a radiolucent pad.
- Centre to the head of the 3rd metacarpal.

Alternative projections

When projections of both hands are required for comparison, e.g. for rheumatoid arthritis, the patient dose is reduced by imaging both hands on one IR with one exposure.

PA for both hands
- Patient seated with elbows flexed.
- Place hands, palmar surface down, onto IR.
- Fingers extended, separated and the thumbs adducted to avoid superimposition.
- Centre midway between both hands at the level of the head of the 3rd metacarpal.

AP oblique for both hands (ball catcher)
- Both forearms and hands in supination with dorsa of hands touching IR.
- Hands internally rotated through 30° and supported on radiolucent pads.
- Fingers extended, separated and the thumbs abducted to avoid superimposition.

- Centre midway between both hands at the level of the head of the 5th metacarpal.

Additional projection

To demonstrate displacement in the event of a fracture or the site of a foreign body.

Lateral
- From the PA position externally rotate the hand through 90° onto the ulnar surface.
- Extend 2nd to 5th digits and ensure that they are superimposed.
- Adjust the thumb to lie at right angles to the palm.
- Centre to the head of the 2nd metacarpal.

Heart (see Chest)

Hip

Basic projections GRID BROAD FOCUS

AP FFD 115cm 35 X 43 CM

- Patient supine with the hip under examination central to the IR in the grid device.

- ASIS parallel to the IR to ensure that there is no rotation of the pelvis.
- Internally rotate both legs through 15–20° to ensure that the entire femoral neck is demonstrated.
- Rest great toes together with the heels apart.
- Centre 2.5 cm distal to a line drawn perpendicular to the midpoint of a line between the ASIS and the symphysis pubis.

Lateral oblique
- From the supine position rotate the patient 45° towards the affected side and support with pads.
- Flex the affected hip and rotate externally until the lateral aspect of the thigh is in contact with the table top.
- Ensure that the contralateral leg does not obscure the ROI.
- Place the top of the IR in the grid device to the ASIS.
- Centre to the crease of the groin in the midline of the femur.

Alternative projection

Where there is a suspected fracture of the hip, a radiograph of the full pelvis should be performed as the initial examination. If there is external rotation and/or shortening of the limb under investigation (clinical indications of a fractured neck of femur), medial rotation of the limb should not be attempted.

AP (both hips)
- Patient supine with the MSP in the midline of the IR in the grid device.
- ASIS equidistant from the IR to ensure that there is no rotation of the pelvis.
- Internally rotate both legs through 15–20° to ensure that the entire femoral neck is demonstrated.
- Rest great toes together with the heels apart.
- Centre to the MSP 2.5 cm above the upper border of the symphysis pubis.

Alternative projection

To demonstrate a true lateral of the hip when patient condition does not allow rotatation onto the affected side.

Horizontal beam lateral
- With patient supine, carefully place a pad under the affected hip to raise it above the mattress.
- Flex the knee of the unaffected limb and elevate the foot.

- Support the raised limb and ensure that there is no rotation of the pelvis.
- The vertical gridded IR is positioned so that it is pushed well into the affected side of the patient just above the iliac crest.
- The IR is adjusted so that it is parallel to the neck of the femur and supported in position.
- Centre a horizontal beam perpendicular to the IR to enter the neck of femur and emerge at the greater trochanter.

Alternative projection

When projections of both hips are required for comparison, e.g. for congenital dysplasia of the hip (CDH), the patient dose is reduced by imaging both on one IR with one exposure. However, the following projection is difficult to achieve other than with young patients.

Lateral oblique of both hips (frog lateral)
- Patient supine with the MSP in the midline of the IR in the grid device.
- ASIS equidistant from the IR to ensure that there is no rotation of the pelvis.
- Flex the hips and knees until the feet are flat on the x-ray table top.

- Abduct the patient's thighs until the soles of the feet are touching and both thighs are at an angle of approximately 30° to the IR.
- Centre 2.5 cm above the upper border of the symphysis pubis in the MSP.

Humerus

When the entire length of the humerus is to be imaged it is essential to include both the shoulder and elbow joint on the resultant images.

Basic projections

For patient comfort these projections are best obtained with the patient in the erect position.

AP 100cm　　Fine Focus　24x30cm

- Patient erect facing the tube.
- Rotate the patient slightly towards the affected side.
- Abduct the arm and supinate the hand until the epicondyles of the humerus are equidistant from the IR.
- Centre to the midpoint of the humerus.
- Exposure on suspended respiration.

Lateral 100cm Fine focus 24×30cm

- Patient facing the IR in the vertical holder.
- Affected arm is abducted with the elbow flexed and the hand placed across the abdomen.
- Trunk rotated away from the affected side to bring the whole of the affected humerus into contact with the IR and the humeral epicondyles superimposed.
- Centre to the midpoint of the humerus.
- Exposure on arrested respiration.

Alternative projections

Where the erect position is not practicable, the patient can be radiographed in the supine position.

AP
- Patient supine and rotated slightly towards the affected side.
- Abduct the arm and supinate the hand until the epicondyles of the humerus are equidistant from the IR.
- Centre to the midpoint of the humerus.
- Exposure on suspended respiration.

Lateral
- From the AP position rotate the humerus medially through 90°.

- Flex the elbow, abduct the arm and internally rotate the hand.
- The medial aspect of the elbow should be in contact with the IR.
- Centre to the midpoint of the humerus.
- Exposure on arrested respiration.

NB: This projection may not produce an image that is at 90° to the AP as the required rotation of the arm may not be achievable.

Hyoid (see Foreign bodies; Thoracic inlet)

Hysterosalpingography

Assessment of the non-gravid uterus under fluoroscopic control. Indications include infertility investigations, recurrent miscarriages, post reversal of sterilisation/ tubal surgery or assessment of caesarean section uterine scar.

Patient preparation

Abstinence from coitus is advised during the period between booking of the appointment and the examination to ensure that there is no chance of pregnancy. The examination should take place between the 4th and 10th day post menstruation as this is generally a few days before ovulation occurs, so reducing the risk of irradiating a recently fertilised ovum. Clear and careful explanation of the procedure to the patient is required as discomfort can occur as a result of the instrumentation used. Apprehensive patients may require premedication, the bladder and rectum must be empty and a muscle relaxant may be given to prevent muscle spasm.

Technique

A preliminary coned radiograph of the pelvic cavity is carried out. The patient is placed in the lithotomy position with the knees flexed over leg rests. Following the insertion of a vaginal speculum the cervix and vagina are cleansed. Using aseptic techniques a cannula is inserted into the cervical canal and the water-soluble contrast agent is introduced slowly into the uterine cavity under fluoroscopic control. The contrast medium can be high-osmolar or low-osmolar (300 mg/ml) with a volume of up to 10–20 ml introduced in stages. Spot films coned to the ROI are taken as the fallopian (uterine) tubes fill and as peritoneal spill occurs. As the gonads are being directly imaged, all measures should be taken to keep the radiation dose to the patient to the absolute minimum.

Patient aftercare

The patient should be advised that vaginal bleeding may occur for a few days and pain may be experienced for up to 2 weeks post examination.

Ilium (see Pelvis; Sacroiliac joints)

Intercondylar notch (see Knee)

Interphalangeal joint (see Fingers; Hand)

Internal auditory meatus (see Petrous temporal bones; Skull)

Intraoral dental radiography (see Bitewing radiography; Occlusal radiography; Periapical radiography)

Intravenous urography

An investigation of the urinary tract following the injection of an intravenous contrast medium.

Patient preparation

Differing patient conditions dictate the preparation of the patient. Those patients with multiple myeloma, diabetes or high uric acid levels are at an increased risk of contrast medium-induced renal failure and therefore should not be dehydrated. A low-residue diet is recommended for 1–2 days prior to the examination so bowel preparation is not normally necessary. However, it is preferable that the patient is ambulant prior to the examination to disperse any bowel gas present. Patients must empty their bladder immediately prior to the examination to prevent dilution of the contrast medium with urine.

Basic projections in the adult patient

A preliminary AP projection of the abdomen is carried out to demonstrate the location and contour of the kidneys and the presence of any obvious renal calculi, to identify any bowel gas patterns which may obscure the renal tract and to establish that the exposure factors are optimum. If the entire renal tract is not demonstrated on a single projection an additional AP projection of the bladder region (*see* Bladder) is carried out.

Following the injection of approximately 50 ml of an intravenous contrast medium a series of projections are performed. Departments have varying protocols for the series taken. A suggested routine would be:

- an immediate coned projection of the renal area, a nephrogram, to demonstrate the renal outlines (in expiration)
- at 5 minutes, a coned projection to demonstrate contrast in the calyceal system (in expiration)
- at 10 minutes, a coned projection of the renal area to demonstrate the pelvis of the kidney well filled (in expiration)

- at 15–20 minutes, a full length AP abdomen to demonstrate the whole of the urinary system (in inspiration)
- post micturition, a coned projection of the bladder area to demonstrate bladder function.

NB: Projections taken on inspiration, expiration and the oblique position are useful for demonstrating relationships between any opacities. They can also highlight any filling defects of the renal tract.

Compression may be applied to the distal ends of the ureters to inhibit the flow of contrast medium from the renal pelvis to the bladder. This is generally applied after the 5-minute coned renal area projection has been performed. The aim is to distend the pelvicalyceal systems to demonstrate any filling defects. This is released immediately prior to the full length abdomen in an attempt to visualise the flow of contrast down the ureters and into the bladder. Compression should not be applied in patients with suspected renal colic, an aortic aneurysm, an abdominal mass or a colostomy, or if there is renal trauma.

Additional projections

- A prone abdominal projection can aid visualisation in cases of ureteric obstruction.
- In cases of suspected renal hypertension a sequence of images taken in rapid succession can evaluate differential rates of contrast excretion.
- If the renal area is obscured by gas, a tomogram of the region may be performed.
- Where ureteric obstruction is demonstrated, films may be performed up to 24 hours post injection to identify any delayed filling of the system.

NB: Relevant markers should be placed on the IRs to record the variations in technique between radiographs.

Additional modalities

- CT is useful when there is suspected trauma or renal mass.
- US can be used as an aid to drainage procedures of e.g. renal cysts. It is often the modality of choice for investigations of the bladder.
- RNI for the evaluation of renal function and assessment of renal transplant rejection.

- Retrograde urography evaluates the collecting system but provides little information as to the physiological capabilities of the urinary system.
- Urethrography to demonstrate urethral strictures.
- Cystography to demonstrate retrograde filling of the lower urinary tract.

Paediatric technique

US or RNI is often the preferred imaging option. If an IVU is necessary a modified technique may be employed limiting the projections taken and therefore the radiation dose received. Bowel preparation is not carried out and a dose of low-osmolar or non-ionic contrast medium is administered intravenously by bodyweight. The limited series of projections, generally a full length AP abdomen, coned to the urinary tract, is carried out but the series is often dictated by departmental protocols. Should the renal area be obscured by faecal matter the administration of a carbonated drink or a proprietary effervescent powder prior to the examination will distend the stomach and often provides good visualisation of the upper urinary tract through its gas-filled outline.

Ischium (see Pelvis)

Jugular foramina (see *also* Skull)

Basic projection
To show both sides with one exposure.

Modified submentovertical (SMV)
- Patient supine or erect at least 30 cm away from the IR.
- Hyperextend the neck until the vertex of the skull rests on the grid device.
- MSP perpendicular to and interpupillary line parallel to the plane of the IR.
- CR angled 20° caudally.
- Centre midway between the EAMs.
- Use close collimation.

Knee

Basic projections
AP 100cm Fine focus 18x24cm
- Patient supine/sitting with affected leg extended and no rotation of the pelvis.
- Place knee directly onto IR.
- Rotate leg approximately 5° internally to ensure femoral epicondyles are equidistant

from the IR and the patella is parallel to the IR and centralised over the femur.
- Centre to the knee joint 2.5 cm below the apex of the patella.

Lateral 100CM FINE FOCUS 18×24CM

Flexion of the knee to a consistent angle is essential for establishing patella alta or patella baja.

- Patient rotated to the affected side with hip slightly flexed, knee flexed by 30°–45° and heel supported on a radiolucent pad.
- Lateral aspect of the knee resting on the IR with the femoral condyles superimposed and patella at 90° to IR.
- Contralateral leg positioned behind affected leg to avoid occluding the ROI.
- Centre to the superior border of the medial tibial condyle.

NB: Acute flexion of the knee will result in the patella being drawn into close contact with the femoral sulcus, preventing adequate demonstration of the patellofemoral joint.

Alternative projection

To better demonstrate genu valgum/varum, to assess joint space narrowing under weight-bearing conditions or as preoperative planning for patients receiving prostheses. Both knees are included on one exposure.

Weight-bearing AP

- Patient erect with posterior aspect of knees in contact with vertical IR.
- Weight distributed evenly between feet.
- Rotate legs approximately 10° internally to ensure that the divergent beam will produce a true AP projection.
- Centre between the knees 2.5 cm below the apices of the patellae.

Alternative projection

To demonstrate a true lateral of the knee when patient condition does not allow rotation onto the affected side.

Horizontal beam lateral

- With patient supine, carefully place a pad under the affected knee to raise it above the mattress.
- To prevent flexion of the affected knee, support the heel on a similar sized radiolucent pad.
- Ensure that the femoral condyles are super-imposed and patella is perpendicular to IR.
- The vertical IR is positioned against the medial aspect of the affected knee and supported in position.

- Centre a horizontal beam perpendicular to the IR to enter the lateral aspect of the knee at the level of the superior border of the tibial condyle.

NB: This projection is also valuable in demonstrating lipohaemarthrosis in trauma patients.

Additional projection

To demonstrate loose bodies within the knee joint.

Intercondylar notch (tunnel)
- Patient prone with affected knee on IR.
- Flex knee until tibia lies at 45° to the IR and support.
- Adjust patient position to centralise patella over the femur.
- To demonstrate the anterior portion of the notch direct a CR angled 45° caudally to the IR to enter the centre of the crease of the knee.
- To demonstrate the posterior portion of the notch direct a CR angled 65° caudally to the IR to enter the centre of the crease of the knee.

Alternative projection

If the patient is unable to achieve the prone position, images can be obtained in the AP position.

- Patient seated with affected knee flexed to produce an angle of 120° between the tibia and femur.
- IR supported on a radiolucent pad under, and in contact with, the distal femur and proximal tibia.
- Ensure that the femoral condyles are equidistant from IR and centralise patella over the femur.
- To demonstrate the anterior portion of the notch direct a CR angled cranially until it is 110° to the long axis of the tibia to enter immediately below the apex of the patella.
- To demonstrate the posterior portion of the notch direct a CR angled cranially until it is 90° to the long axis of the tibia to enter immediately below the apex of the patella.

NB: This projection results in the primary beam being directed towards the gonads, so gonad protection must be used.

Additional projection

To demonstrate the patellofemoral joint surface and the congruence of the patella within the femoral sulcus. This view should *not* be attempted in patients suffering patellar trauma.

Alternative projection

Inferosuperior
- Patient prone with affected knee flexed by 60°.
- Support vertical lower leg with radiolucent pads.
- Patella centralised over the femur.
- IR placed under the distal femur.
- Angle the CR 15° cranially.
- Centre to the apex of the patella.
- Displace the IR until it is centred to the CR.

Inferosuperior (skyline)
- Patient supine/sitting with affected hip flexed and knee flexed by 45°.
- Patient holds the IR with the lower edge in contact with the superior aspect of the lower femur at 90° to the long axis of the patella.
- Angle the CR 10° cranially.
- Centre to the apex of the patella.
- Adjust the IR until it is perpendicular and centred to the CR.

NB: As the CR is directed at the trunk in this projection, gonad protection should be used.

Larynx (see Foreign bodies; Thoracic inlet)

Lumbar vertebrae

Basic projections *long axis body to the long axis of body*

The sacroiliac joints should be included in this
projection. *Broad focus*

AP   FFD 100   30×40cm IR in Grid

- Patient supine with MSP aligned to the
  centre of the IR in the grid device.
- Flex hips and knees until soles of the feet are
  resting on the table to reduce lumbar lordosis.
- Centre to the MSP at the lower costal margin.
- Exposure on arrested expiration.

30 × 40cm BROAD

Lateral   FFD 150cm due to OFD

- Patient lies in left lateral position with the
  MSP parallel to the IR.
- The mid-coronal plane is aligned to the
  centre of the IR in the grid device.
- Arms on the pillow, knees and hips flexed to
  stabilise.
- A radiolucent pad under the waist may be
  necessary if palpation of the spinous
  processes reveals that the long axis of the
  spine is not parallel to the IR.

- Centre at the level of the lower costal margin (LCM), 7.5–10 cm anterior to the spinous process of L3.
- Exposure on arrested expiration.

NB: The left lateral projection is usually performed unless there is a right lumbar scoliosis present. This uses the liver to reduce the dose to the more radiosensitive organs on the left side of the abdomen.

Additional projections

To demonstrate the pars interarticularis and the articular processes of the lumbar vertebrae.

Right posterior oblique (RPO)
- From the AP position, rotate the patient 45° to the right and support with pads.
- MSP aligned to the centre of the IR in the grid device.
- Centre 5 cm medial to the ASIS of the raised side at the level of the LCM.
- Exposure on arrested expiration.

LPO
- From the AP position, rotate the patient 45° to the left and support with pads.
- MSP aligned to the centre of the IR in the grid device.

- Centre 5 cm medial to the ASIS of the raised side at the level of the LCM.
- Exposure on arrested expiration.

NB: Both these projections demonstrate the articular processes closest to the IR.

Additional projection

Lateral lumbosacral junction
- Position the patient as for the lateral lumbar spine.
- Centre 7.5 cm anterior to the spinous process of L5.
- A tube angle of 5° caudally can also be used.
- Exposure on arrested respiration.

Lungs (see Chest)

Mammography

Visualisation of the breast to confirm/deny the presence of abnormalities within the glandular tissues. Mammography is a challenging technique requiring specialised skills as breasts vary considerably in size, shape and mobility, with each examination tailored to meet the specific needs of individual patients.

Women who attend for mammography fall into two distinct categories:

- symptomatic women who require accurate information that will aid in the definitive diagnosis of their condition
- asymptomatic women who attend as part of the National Health Service Breast Screening Programme (NHSBSP). The NHSBSP offers free breast screening approximately every 3 years to women within the highest incidence range for breast cancer, between 50 and 70 years of age. Once beyond this age, women can self-refer.

The routine projections carried out on both groups of women are the same and require the use of dedicated mammography imaging equipment and processing facilities. The breast has inherently low radiographic contrast and therefore the kVp range utilised is well below that used in conventional radiography, typically 28–31 kVp.

Techniques vary but image criteria with regard to the resultant image are critical. The density range of the resultant images must be between 1.4 and 1.8 to maximise visualisation of any minute areas of calcification present which can be indicative of a developing carcinoma. Very small changes in the breast may be the only indication that there is breast disease present so optimum image quality is essential. In order to obtain images of the highest quality, equipment must be rigorously maintained in order to operate within the very specific parameters required for breast imaging.

Basic projections

Craniocaudal (CC)

- Patient stands/sits facing the tube, shoulders relaxed, head turned away from the side under investigation and placed against face guard.
- The hand of the side under investigation should hold the support handle on the mammography unit.
- Standing to the medial aspect of the breast to be imaged, lift the breast to its maximum height at the inframammary fold.
- Position the grid device at this level.
- Patient leaning well into the machine, gently pull the breast tissue onto the grid device, ensuring that the axillary border and medial aspect of the breast are included.
- Nipple must be in profile.
- Immobilise the breast with one hand, maintaining the maximum amount of breast tissue on the IR; apply compression gently and as the compression paddle

descends, slide the hand that is maintaining the breast in position towards the nipple; continue to apply compression until the breast is taut.

NB: Both sides are taken for comparison.

45° Mediolateral oblique (MLO) (right breast)

- From the vertical position the tube is rotated until the grid device forms an angle of 45° with the floor and 45° with the axillary side of the breast.
- Patient stands/sits facing the x-ray machine with the lateral border of the thorax alongside and slightly medial to the grid device.
- The height of the machine is set provisionally to bring the top of the grid device to the level of axilla.
- Standing to the left side of the patient, take the right breast in the left hand and lift the maximum amount of breast tissue forward and away from the chest wall.
- The right upper humerus is supported in the right hand; the patient is asked to lean forwards and laterally to place the axilla into the corner of the grid device.
- Nipple should be in profile.
- Inframammary angle included in ROI and no skin folds present.

- The pectoral muscle is included down to nipple level across the IR at an angle of 20–35° from vertical.
- Adequate compression is slowly applied until the breast is held firmly in a position that best achieves an even thickness of breast tissue across the entire breast from nipple to chest wall yet is tolerable to the patient.
- Exposure on arrested respiration. Release compression immediately after the exposure has taken place.

NB: This projection, when performed correctly, will demonstrate the majority of the breast tissue on one film.

45° MLO (left breast)

- Reverse of right breast.

Additional modalities

- US is useful for the demonstration of cystic lesions within the breast tissue and can be used to guide fine-needle aspirations and drainage procedures.
- MRI is highly sensitive to small abnormalities, can image breast implants and ruptures, is effective in imaging dense breasts and determines if tumour invasion

to the chest wall has occurred. It has the disadvantages of high cost, limited availability and dependence on the use of contrast media, and it is more time-consuming than mammography.

Mandible

Basic projections

PA
- Patient erect facing the IR in a vertical grid device.
- Nose and forehead in contact with midline of grid device.
- MSP and radiographic baseline perpendicular to the IR.
- Centre to the MSP between the angles of the mandible, approximately 7.5 cm below the inion (external occipital protruberance).

Lateral oblique
To demonstrate the mandibular ramus

- Patient supine or erect with the affected side towards the IR; no grid is required.
- Slightly raise the chin.
- From the lateral position tilt the head towards the IR.

- Tube angled 10° cranially until the MSP makes an angle of 15° with the IR.
- Centre 5 cm below the angle of the mandible remote from the IR.

Lateral mandible
- Patient seated facing the IR.
- Head rotated through 90° to place affected side against IR.
- MSP parallel to IR.
- Raise chin slightly.
- Centre to the angle of the mandible with a horizontal CR.

Mastoids (see also Skull)

CT has all but replaced plain radiographs of the mastoid area.

Basic projections

Fronto-occipital (FO) 35° caudal
- Patient supine or erect.
- MSP perpendicular to and centred to the IR in the grid device.
- Radiographic baseline perpendicular to the IR.
- Tube angled 35° caudally.

- Centre to the MSP at the level of the EAMs.
- Use close collimation.

SMV

- Patient supine or erect at least 30 cm away from the IR.
- Hyperextend the neck until the vertex of the skull rests on the grid device.
- MSP perpendicular to and interpupillary line parallel to the plane of the IR.
- Centre to the MSP between the EAMs.
- Use close collimation.

Lateral oblique

- With the patient in the erect position, turn the head to bring the affected side closer to the IR in the grid device.
- MSP parallel to and interpupillary line perpendicular to the IR.
- Fold the pinna of the ear nearest the IR forward to avoid soft tissue shadowing.
- CR 25° caudally.
- Centre 5 cm superior and posterior to the raised EAM.
- Use close collimation.

Profile of mastoid process

- Patient in the FO position.
- Radiographic baseline is perpendicular to the IR.

- Rotate the head 35° away from the side of interest until the process is in profile.
- Tube angled 15° caudally.
- Centre directly over the mastoid process under examination.

Maxilla (see Facial bones)

Mediastinum (see Chest)

Nasal bones (see *also* Facial bones)

Plain radiological investigation of the nasal bones is no longer routine as even positive findings do not influence patient management[3].

Non-accidental injury (see Skeletal survey)

Occlusal radiography

Basic projection

To demonstrate the upper anterior teeth and the anterior part of the maxilla using intraoral dental x-ray equipment and a packet occlusal IR.

Upper maxillary occlusal
- Patient seated with head supported.
- Occlusal plane parallel to the floor.
- IR is placed centrally with its long axis crosswise onto the occlusal surface of the teeth (with children the long axis will be placed anteroposteriorly).
- The x-ray tube side of the IR is uppermost.
- Patient bites teeth together gently to avoid artefacts on the resultant image.
- The x-ray tube head is positioned above the patient.
- Aiming downwards with an angle of 65–70° to the IR, the central ray enters the patient in the midline through the bridge of the nose.

Alternative projection

To demonstrate the floor of the mouth and the tooth-bearing part of the mandible.

Lower mandibular 90° occlusal
- Occlusal IR is placed centrally with its long axis crosswise onto the occlusal surface of the teeth.
- The x-ray tube side of the IR faces downwards.
- Patient bites teeth together gently to avoid artefacts on the resultant image.

- The chin is raised as far as is comfortable and the head supported.
- The x-ray tubehead is positioned below the patient's chin.
- The central ray enters the patient in the midline at the level of the first molars at 90° to the IR.

Odontoid process (see Cervical vertebrae)

Oesophagus (see Barium swallow; Foreign bodies)

Olecranon process (see *also* Elbow)

The forearm and humerus will appear superimposed on these views but the olecranon process can be seen in profile.

Basic projection

To demonstrate the articular margin of the olecranon and humerus.

Inferosuperior (axial)

- The elbow and shoulder joints should be in the same horizontal plane.

- Place the fully flexed elbow onto the IR.
- Humeral epicondyles equidistant from IR.
- Place the palm of the hand facing the shoulder.
- Centre 5 cm superior to the olecranon process.

Alternative projection

To demonstrate the dorsum of the olecranon and the olecranon fossa.

AP axial 20°

- The elbow and shoulder joints should be in the same horizontal plane.
- Place the fully flexed elbow onto the IR.
- Epicondyles equidistant from IR.
- Place the palm of the hand facing the shoulder.
- Angle the tube 20° cranially.
- Centre 5 cm superior to the olecranon process.

Optic foramen (see *also* Skull)

Basic projection

PA oblique

- Patient PA erect or prone with MSP centred to the IR in the grid device.

- From the occipitofrontal (OF) position adjust the head until the radiographic baseline is at 35° to the IR.
- Rotate the head through 45°, placing the orbit of interest to the centre of the IR.
- CR to pass through the orbit nearest the IR.

Orbit (see Facial bones; Foreign bodies; Skull)

Orthopantomography (OPT, OPG)
(see Dental panoramic tomography)

Paranasal sinuses

The following projections provide limited evidence in the diagnosis of pathology, and are mainly used to identify fluid collection or fractures.

Basic projections

To demonstrate the maxillary sinuses.

OM
- Patient PA erect with MSP centred to the IR in a vertical grid device.
- Chin and nose in contact with the centre of the grid device.

- MSP perpendicular to IR with EAMs equidistant from it.
- Adjust the head until the radiographic baseline is 45° above the horizontal plane.
- Centre to the MSP above the inion to exit at the level of the lower orbital margin.

NB: The sphenoid and ethmoid sinuses will be demonstrated if the patient has an open mouth whilst the exposure is made.

OF 15°
- Patient PA erect with MSP centred to the IR in a vertical grid device.
- Forehead and nose in contact with the centre of the grid device.
- MSP perpendicular to IR with EAMs equidistant from it.
- Adjust head until the radiographic baseline is 15° above the horizontal plane.
- Centre to the MSP in the occipital region to exit at the level of the nasion.

Lateral
- Patient PA erect facing vertical grid device.
- Rotate the head towards the affected side until the MSP is parallel to the IR and the interpupillary line perpendicular to the IR.

- Centre 2.5 cm behind the outer canthus of the eye along the radiographic baseline.

Additional modalities

- CT is commonly used to identify disease of the paranasal sinuses and for preoperative assessment prior to endoscopic surgery.
- MRI is a valuable tool in providing information regarding tumours, invasion and bony destruction.

Parotid gland (see Sialography)

Pars interarticularis (see Lumbar vertebrae)

Patella (see *also* Knee)

Although the patella is demonstrated on a basic AP knee radiograph, there is an element of distortion due to the large SID. A PA projection gives better resolution, but may be unacceptable to the patient.

Basic projections

PA 100CM Fine Focus 18X24CM

- Patient prone with affected leg extended.
- IR placed under the affected knee.
- Leg adjusted to bring patella parallel to IR and centralised on femur.
- Support ankle on pad for comfort.
- Centre to the patella.

Inferosuperior
- As for knee.

Lateral
- As for knee.

Pelvimetry

The radiographic examination of the gravid pelvis in order for obstetricians to decide the need for a caesarean section is no longer appropriate and should not be undertaken.[3]

Alternative modalities

- MRI pelvimetry is now the method of choice to avoid the ionising radiation dose to both patient and baby.

- Although a high-dose modality, limited imaging of the pelvic area using CT provides more accurate measurements at a lower dose than plain film pelvimetry.

Pelvis

LMP = LAST MENSTRAL PERIOD.

Basic projection

AP 115cm FFD 35×43cm BROAD focus

- Patient supine with MSP aligned to the centre of the IR in the grid device.
- Extend and medially rotate the legs until the heels are slightly apart and the great toes touching to bring the femoral necks parallel to the IR.
- MSP perpendicular to IR and ASIS equidistant from it.
- Centre to the MSP 5 cm above the symphysis pubis.

NB: External rotation and shortening of the injured limb is a clear clinical indication of a fractured neck of femur and medial rotation of the limb should not be attempted.

Percutaneous transhepatic cholangiogram (PTC) (see Biliary tract)

Periapical radiography

Periapical radiography techniques provide information on individual teeth, the associated alveolar bone and the tissues surrounding the apices. To achieve optimum images the tooth and IR should be in as close contact as possible, and be parallel to each other, with the central ray at right angles to both. Periapical radiography can be performed using either the paralleling technique or the bisecting angle technique. Projections should be carried out using the paralleling technique where possible as recommended by the National Radiological Protection Board (1994)[4] and in their 2001 Guidance notes for dental practitioners.[5]

Although this technique can be uncomfortable for the patient due to the bulky IR holders or digital sensors used, it has distinct advantages. When all the positioning devices are used correctly, irrespective of the position of the patient's head, the images produced show little magnification, minimal elongation/foreshortening of the periapical tissues, good periodontal bone levels and the crowns of the teeth. The resultant radiographs are also reproducible due to the fact that the positions of the x-ray beam, teeth and IR are fixed and remain relative to each other. There are a number of proprietary holders available for the paralleling technique. They consist of a holder for the IR which keeps it parallel to the teeth, a bite block and an x-ray beam aiming device. There are anterior holders for imaging the maxillary and mandibular incisors and canines and posterior holders for imaging the maxillary and mandibular premolars and molars. Selection of the correct holder is essential: they must not be interchanged or incorrect centring will occur.

- For incisors and canines and an IR of 22 × 35 mm is used and for premolars and molars an IR 31 × 41 mm is used.
- The patient is seated and head supported.
- The appropriate IR is placed with the tube-side facing the lingual surface of the teeth in the appropriate holder and placed in the mouth as described below.
- In all regions the patient is required to close their mouth over the holder and bite to retain the IR in position.

- The beam is aligned to the centre of the beam-indicating device on the holder and the central ray will be directed to the centre of the tooth or teeth under examination at a point level with the gum margin.

Upper incisors and canines
- IR with short axis into holder behind each tooth to be examined and far enough into the oral cavity for the palate to accommodate its height.

Upper premolars and molars
- Long axis of IR into holder with midpoint of teeth under examination centred on the IR.

Lower incisors
- Place IR with short axis into holder.
- Use cotton wool roll to ease placement of the IR which needs to be positioned under the tongue.

Lower canines
- Place IR with short axis into holder.
- Use cotton wool roll between biting block and the crowns of the teeth to ease placement of IR into lingual sulcus.
- This is an area where parallelism is difficult to obtain as a slight angle between the teeth

and film may occur with a gap between the centrally situated canine and the IR.

Lower premolars
- Place IR with long axis into holder.
- As IR is placed under the tongue a small gap between it and the premolars is unavoidable.
- Midpoint of teeth under examination centred on the IR.

Lower molars
- Place IR with long axis into holder.
- The lower third molar can be difficult to image so if the anterior corner of the IR is placed to the edge of the bite block it is possible to place the IR in contact with the mandible behind the molar region and increase the success in imaging this tooth.

Only when patient condition or the anatomy of the mouth makes the use of this technique unfeasible should the bisecting angle technique be employed. This technique is more comfortable for the patient but is very operator dependent and patient positioning is critical to its success. To produce an acceptable image, the IR is positioned as close as possible to the affected tooth without it being bent. The angle between the long axis of the tooth and the long axis of the IR is gauged and, as the name of the technique suggests, is bisected. As the degree of angulation required to image each individual tooth will vary with anatomical differences, great skill is required by the operator to produce an image that is not distorted. Reproducibility is an issue because of the many variables involved. Standardising patient position provides a baseline to measure and control vertical angulation and aids the centring of the x-ray beam as it orientates the tooth in a vertical position and indicates the apex of the tooth.

Like the paralleling technique there are IR holders available for use or the patient is asked to support the IR using their index finger or thumb.

- To image the maxillary teeth the head is positioned so that a line from the ala of the nose to the tragus of the ear is parallel to the floor.
- To image the mandibular teeth the head is positioned so that a line drawn from the angle of the mouth to the tragus of the ear, is parallel to the floor.

- The MSP is perpendicular to the floor for both projections.
- When the IR is positioned and supported in place by the patient's finger, approximately 2 mm should extend beyond the occlusal or incisor edges.
- The CR should be centred to the tooth under examination with all centring points lying on the same plane, i.e. for maxillary teeth the ala–tragal line, and for mandibular teeth 1 cm above the lower border of the mandible.
- CR directed at right angles to the bisection of the tooth and the film. It should be noted that the angle between the individual tooth and the film rises gradually from molar to incisor regions so the angle of the CR will increase.
- In the lower 3rd molar region, the film and tooth are usually parallel so the x-ray beam can be horizontal.

NB: The angle between a tooth and the film is dependent on the height of the dome of the palate or the depth of the floor of the mouth.

Diagnostic images should be obtained using a film of speed E or F to keep radiation dose to the patient to a minimum.

The film should be orientated in the mouth with the 'dot' to the crown of the teeth so that it does not obscure the apices.

Petrous portion of the temporal bones (see *also* Skull)

There are numerous projections that can be used to demonstrate the petrous part of the temporal bones, but these have been superseded by the ease of use of CT techniques.

Basic projections

FO 35° caudal
- Patient supine or erect.
- MSP perpendicular to and centred to the IR in the grid device.
- Radiographic baseline perpendicular to the IR.
- Tube angled 35° caudally.
- Centre to the MSP at the level of the EAMs.
- Use close collimation.

Perorbital
- Patient PA erect or prone with MSP perpendicular and centred to the IR in the grid device.

- Adjust head until the radiographic baseline is perpendicular to the IR.
- CR to pass through the MSP to emerge between the orbits.
- Use close collimation.

PA oblique to demonstrate IAMs (Stenver's)
- Patient PA erect or prone with forehead and nose in contact with the grid device.
- Orbit of side of interest centred to the IR.
- Adjust head until the radiographic baseline is perpendicular to the IR.
- Rotate the head until the MSP is at 45° to the IR.
- Tube angled 12° cranially.
- Centre midway between the visible EAM and the external occipital protuberance (EOP).

SMV
- Patient supine or erect at least 30 cm away from the IR.
- Hyperextend the neck until the vertex of the skull rests on the grid device.
- MSP perpendicular to and interpupillary line parallel to the plane of the IR.
- Centre to the MSP between the EAMs.
- Use close collimation.

Pharynx (see Foreign bodies; Thoracic inlet)

Pituitary fossa (see *also* Skull)

Localised views of the pituitary fossa (sella turcica) with close collimation have largely been replaced by CT or MRI.

Basic projections

FO 30° caudal (coned)
- Patient supine or erect.
- MSP perpendicular to and centred to the IR in the grid device.
- Radiographic baseline perpendicular to the IR.
- Tube angled 30° caudally.
- Centre to the MSP 5 cm above the glabella.

OF (coned)
- Patient PA erect or prone with MSP centred and perpendicular to the IR in the grid device.
- Adjust head until the radiographic baseline is perpendicular to the IR.
- CR to pass through the MSP to emerge at the glabella.

Lateral (coned)
- Patient erect facing the IR.
- Turn patient's head through 90° to bring the affected side in contact with the IR in the grid device.
- MSP parallel to and interpupillary line perpendicular to the IR.
- Centre 2.5 cm superior and 2.5 cm anterior to the EAM.

SECTION 2

Radial head (see *also* Elbow)

Routine projections of the elbow fail to adequately demonstrate the radial head in its entirety.

Basic projections

AP oblique (external rotation)
- The wrist, elbow and shoulder should be in same horizontal plane as the IR.
- Fully extend elbow joint and supinate hand.
- Rotate the arm laterally from the shoulder joint through 25°.
- Centre over the radial head.

Lateral
- The forearm is placed on the table with the ulnar border of the hand and forearm in contact with the IR.
- Elbow is flexed to 90°.
- The wrist, elbow and shoulder should be in the same horizontal plane as the IR.
- The humeral epicondyles should be superimposed and perpendicular to the IR.
- Centre over the lateral epicondyle of the humerus.
- One exposure is made with the hand in each of the following positions:
  - supinated
  - lateral (thumb up)
  - pronated
  - hand internally rotated.

Additional projection

Position as for lateral elbow and direct a CR with a 45° angulation towards the humerus to the lateral epicondyle of the humerus.

Radius (see Forearm)

Ribs (see *also* Chest)

Oblique projections of the ribs, requested as a result of trauma to a patient, are not always justified as patient management will rarely be affected by diagnosis of a fracture. They are, however, useful in the localisation of metastatic disease.

Basic projections

PA
• As for chest

AP obliques (right or left posterior obliques)
• Patient AP erect, rotated 45° with the affected side closer to the IR.
• Abduct and elevate the arm of the affected side.
• Centre midway between the MSP and the lateral border of the thorax of the side nearest the IR.
• Expose in full inspiration to demonstrate ribs above the diaphragm.
• Expose in full expiration to demonstrate ribs below the diaphragm.

AP (lower ribs)
• Patient erect or supine.
• IR orientated crossways to include both sides.
• Abduct the arms from the body.
• Centre to the MSP at the level of the iliac crests.
• Expose in full expiration.

Rotator cuff (see Shoulder)

Sacroiliac joints (see *also* Lumbar vertebrae)

The sacroiliac joints (SIJs) will be demonstrated on an AP projection of the lumbar spine but the following coned projections will provide better visualisation.

Basic projection IN GRID

PA 100cm BROAD Focus 24x 30cm

• Patient prone with MSP aligned to the centre of the IR in the grid device.
• Tube angled 35° caudally.
• Centre to the MSP at the level of the posterior superior iliac spine (PSIS).
• Exposure on arrested respiration.

NB: The obliquity of the sacroiliac joints in the prone position is parallel to the diverging beam, thus demonstrating both joints with one exposure.

Additional projections

Posterior obliques
- Patient supine with MSP aligned to the centre of the IR in the grid device.
- Elevate the side under investigation by 25° and support trunk in this position.
- Centre 2.5 cm medially to the raised ASIS.
- Repeat for contralateral SIJ.

Sacrum

Basic projections   *24 × 30 cm*

AP *1000M BROAD/FINE FOCUS*
- Patient supine with MSP aligned to the centre of the IR in the grid device.
- CR angled 15° cranially.
- Centre to the MSP 5 cm above the symphysis pubis.

Lateral *1000M BROAD FOCUS*   *24 × 300M*
- Patient lying in the true lateral position.
- Centre midway between the PSIS and sacrococcygeal junction.

NB: Radiation protection for female patients cannot be used on these projections and, therefore, the request should be carefully considered if the patient is of childbearing age.

Salivary glands (see Sialography)

Scaphoid

Each department will have its own series of projections for the scaphoid, but the following are the most common. Some scaphoid fractures are not demonstrated on initial radiographs and will require delayed images after 10–14 days in order to assess any bone resorption.

Basic projections 24 × 30

PA in ulnar deviation 100cm fine focus
- Patient seated with elbow flexed.
- Place wrist and distal forearm onto IR.
- Without moving the forearm, the patient moves the fingers laterally until the wrist is in extreme ulnar deviation.
- Centre to the scaphoid.

PA oblique
- From the PA position rotate the hand 45° towards the lateral border.
- Support the wrist with a pad.
- Centre to the scaphoid.

Lateral
- From the PA position rotate the hand externally 90° to the lateral position.
- Rotate the wrist another 5° laterally to ensure that the styloid processes are superimposed.
- Centre to the scaphoid.

AP oblique
- From the lateral position rotate the hand externally 45°.
- Support the wrist with a pad.
- Centre to the scaphoid.

Additional projection

PA with 45° angulation and ulnar deviation
- Patient seated with elbow flexed.
- Place wrist and distal forearm onto IR.
- Without moving the forearm, the patient moves the fingers laterally until the wrist is in extreme ulnar deviation.
- CR angled 45° towards the elbow.
- Centre to the scaphoid.

Scapula

Basic projections

AP 100cm Fine Focus 24×30cm

- Patient erect/supine and slightly rotated (approximately 30°) towards the affected side to bring the scapula parallel to the IR.
- Abduct the arm and supinate the hand.
- Centre to a point 8 cm below the midpoint of the clavicle.
- Exposure on arrested respiration.

Lateral 100cm Fine Focus 24×30cm

- Patient erect/prone facing the IR.
- Abduct and extend the humerus of the affected side and flex the elbow, resting the arm across the body.
- Rotate the body approximately 30° towards the affected side to bring the blade of the scapula perpendicular to the IR with the shoulder in close contact with the IR.
- Centre to a point just medial to the midpoint of the palpable scapula.

Scoliosis

Radiographs of the whole spine in scoliosis serve several purposes: to confirm the diagnosis; to exclude other pathologies; to allow accurate evaluation of the site and severity of the deformity; to distinguish structural from compensatory curves; to assess skeletal maturity; to allow subsequent monitoring of curve progression, and follow-up of surgical correction. Reproducible radiographs are essential in providing the means for accurate measurements to be made and appropriate patient management to be planned. Routine measurements made from radiographs include the Cobb angle (degree of lateral curve), the axial rotation of the apical vertebrae and the Risser sign (level of fusion of the iliac crests).

Idiopathic scoliosis most often develops in adolescent years and affects more girls than boys. Radiographic imaging usually continues over a considerable length of time and so radiation protection for these developing patients must be a major consideration. Close collimation is extremely difficult to achieve as the iliac crests may need to be imaged and the severity of the curve may require a wide field of view. Breast tissue, the thyroid gland and the gonads may have to be included in the main beam for the initial radiographic examination but breast and gonad shielding can be used in subsequent examinations.

Some departments choose to use a basic PA projection to reduce the primary beam to the breasts and thyroid, while some still use an AP projection. Usually a grid is utilised in the erect bucky, but some departments are now using a non-grid technique to reduce the patient dose. This is thought to be acceptable as the level of detail required to monitor curve progression in follow-up films is reduced.

A large IR (35×90 cm) will need to be used to demonstrate the spine from C7 to the sacrum on one exposure.

Basic projections

AP or PA standing spine

- Patient erect against the IR (PA or AP).
- Shoes removed and weight bearing equally on both feet.
- Arms at the patient's sides.
- Position the IR to include C7 and the whole of the sacrum.
- Centre to the IR in the MSP.
- Exposure on arrested respiration.

NB: If the patient has a known leg-length inequality, another AP/PA projection may be required with them using a compensating block to bring the pelvis level.

Lateral standing spine
- Patient erect with the right side against the IR.
- Shoes removed and weight bearing equally on both feet.
- Arms raised and supported in front at shoulder height, e.g. on drip stand.
- Position the IR to include C7 and the whole of the sacrum.
- Centre to the IR at the mid-axillary line.
- Exposure on arrested respiration.

Additional projections

To demonstrate the flexibility of a curve, usually prior to surgery, lateral bending films may be requested. Primary curves (structural) will not reduce when bending but secondary curves (compensatory) will.

Lateral bending projections
- Patient supine.
- Patient helped to achieve maximal lateral flexion to the right.
- There should be no forward flexion.
- Position the IR to include the sacrum and the upper end-vertebra (at least T5).
- Centre in the MSP to the IR.
- Exposure on arrested respiration.

- Repeat with maximal lateral flexion to the left.

Sella turcica (see Pituitary fossa)

Shoulder

Basic projections

AP *100cm Fine Focus 18x24cm*

- Patient erect/supine, rotated 30° towards the affected side until the scapula is parallel to the IR.
- If the patient is supine, support the raised side on radiolucent pads.
- Slightly abduct the arm and supinate the hand until the limb is in the anatomical position.
- Centre to the humeral head, 2.5 cm below the coracoid process of the scapula.
- Exposure on suspended respiration.

Superoinferior

- Patient seated, affected arm abducted, elbow flexed.
- Lean the patient across the IR until the shoulder joint is central to the IR, hand pronated and resting on the table.

- Tilt the patient's head towards the unaffected shoulder to avoid its superimposition on the resultant image.
- Centre to the head of the humerus.
- A slight angulation towards the elbow may be required if the patient is unable to fully abduct the affected arm.
- Exposure on arrested respiration.

Alternative projection

In cases of acute injury only limited abduction of the arm may be possible.

Inferosuperior
- Patient supine with shoulder slightly raised off the table to ensure all ROI can be imaged.
- Abduct the affected arm to as near 90° as is tolerable and supinate the hand.
- Turn the patient's head away from the affected side.
- Place the vertical IR against the superior border of the shoulder and well into the patient's neck.
- Tube angle of 15° towards the shoulder joint is generally required.
- Centre to the axilla.
- Exposure on suspended respiration.

Alternative projection

To demonstrate dislocation of the shoulder joint when the patient is unable to abduct the affected limb.

'Y' projection

- Patient erect with the anterior surface of the affected limb against a vertical IR holder.
- If patient condition allows, place the back of the hand of the affected limb onto the posterior surface of the hip.
- Rotate the unaffected side 60° away from the IR, bringing the blade of the scapula perpendicular to the IR.
- Centre just medial to the midpoint of the palpable scapula.
- Exposure on arrested respiration.

NB: The Y is formed by the acromion, coracoid process and the body of the scapula. If an anterior dislocation is present, the head of humerus will be beneath the coracoid process. In cases of posterior dislocation the humeral head will be demonstrated beneath the acromion process.

Additional projection

To demonstrate the insertion of the subscapular tendon.

Internal rotation
- Position the patient as for AP shoulder.
- Rotate the affected arm internally and rest the dorsum of the hand on the posterior aspect of the hip.
- Centre 2.5 cm inferior to the coracoid process.
- Exposure on suspended respiration.

Additional projection

To demonstrate the greater tubercle of the humerus and the insertion of the supraspinatus tendon.

External rotation
- Position the patient as for AP shoulder.
- Slightly abduct the arm and supinate the hand until the humeral epicondyles are parallel to the IR.
- Centre 2.5 cm inferior to the coracoid process.
- Exposure on suspended respiration.

Sialography

Examination of the salivary glands and ducts following the injection of a contrast medium. Indications include pain and/or recurrent swelling; contraindications include acute infection or inflammation.

Patient preparation

Remove any radiopaque artefacts. No premedication is generally required. Prior to examination a secretory stimulant can be given. Preliminary projections, of a density adequate to demonstrate the soft tissue structures under investigation, and dictated by the gland under investigation, are carried out.

Approximately 2 ml of a warmed contrast medium, high-osmolar or preferably low-osmolar (240–320 mg/ml), is then injected into the orifice of the duct of the gland under investigation via a fine catheter. If a water-soluble contrast agent is used it is possible to repeat the examination after 15 minutes. This is not the case with an oil-based contrast agent as it is gradually absorbed and the area under examination is obscured.

Following the injection of the contrast medium the preliminary projections are repeated.

A sialogue (a slice of lemon or citric acid) can then be given to the patient and post secretory projections performed if required.

Preliminary and post-injection projections

PA/AP parotid gland
- Patient supine or erect.
- Centre IR to parotid gland.
- Radiographic baseline 90° to the IR.
- Head rotated 5° to the unaffected side.
- Centre midway between symphysis menti and angle of mandible on the side under investigation.
- Collimate to demonstrate the parotid gland lateral to and clear of the ramus of the mandible.

Lateral parotid gland
- Patient supine or erect with the affected side towards the IR.
- Head in a true lateral position with the neck extended.
- Centre 2.5 cm superior to the angle of the mandible.
- Collimate to demonstrate bony structures, soft tissue structures and mandibular rami free of cervical spine.

Lateral oblique parotid gland
- Patient supine or erect with the affected side towards the IR.

- Head in a true lateral position with the neck extended and chin raised.
- Tilt the head towards the IR until the MSP makes an angle of 15° with the IR.
- CR angled 10° cranially.
- Centre 5 cm below the angle of the mandible remote from the IR.
- Collimate to demonstrate bony structures, soft tissue structures and mandibular rami free of cervical spine.

Lateral submandibular gland
- Patient supine or erect with the affected side towards the IR.
- Head in a true lateral position with the neck extended.
- Centre to the inferior margin of the angle of the mandible.
- Depress tongue.
- Exposure on arrested respiration.

Lateral oblique submandibular gland
- Patient supine with the affected side towards the IR.
- From the lateral position tilt the head to the IR until the MSP makes an angle of 15° with the IR.
- CR angled 10° cranially.

• Centre 1 cm anterior to the angle of the mandible remote from the IR.

NB: No grid is required for these projections.

Inferosuperior submandibular gland
• Patient sitting, supine or erect with chin raised and head tilted backwards.
• Shoulders in the same transverse plane.
• Place a correctly orientated dental occlusal IR with the long axis transversely, as far back as the patient will tolerate in the mouth, pushed towards the affected side.
• Instruct the patient to gently close mouth.
• Centre below the mandible to the centre of the IR.

Alternative modalities

• MR sialography. Non-contrast studies are useful in differentiating benign/low-grade malignant from high-grade tumours whilst contrast enhancement is useful in the differential diagnosis of cystic or solid lesions and determining the perineural spread of malignant disease.
• Sialoscintigraphy gives an assessment of salivary gland function and patency.
• Contrast enhanced CT is useful for assessing tumours.

Skeletal survey

Skeletal survey is the radiological investigation in suspected cases of child abuse. The British Society of Paediatric Radiology (BSPR) recommend that it is undertaken in suspected physical non-accidental injury (NAI) in children under 3 years and in siblings of children with proven NAI (also under 3 years). Most departments will have a local protocol for a skeletal survey, but the following list is based on the recommendations of the BSPR.

Basic projections

- Lateral and AP skull (and Townes if appropriate).
- AP chest including clavicles (erect if strong suspicion of lung injury).
- AP abdomen with pelvis and hips.
- Lateral spine (cervical and thoracolumbar).
- AP both forearms and shoulders.
- AP both legs (femora, tibiae and fibulae).
- PA both hands.
- PA both feet.
- Lateral coned projections of knees/ankles/ elbows/wrists (to demonstrate metaphyseal injuries).

NB: A single image (babygram) must be avoided as it gives unsatisfactory projections of the limbs and joints, together with an unsatisfactory exposure for the combined chest, abdomen and pelvis.

Additional projections

- Orthogonal views of any suspected long bone injuries.
- Oblique views of the ribs.
- Follow-up views in 7–10 days in selected cases.

Additional modalities

- CT brain imaged with brain and bone windows will demonstrate a linear skull fracture.
- Interval MRI may give better detail of subdural haematomas and parenchymal injury.

Skull

Basic projections

To demonstrate the cranium.

Fronto-occipital 30° caudal (Townes)
- Patient supine or erect.
- MSP perpendicular to and centred to the IR in the grid device.
- EAMs equidistant from IR.
- Radiographic baseline perpendicular to the IR.
- Tube angled 30° caudally.
- Centre to the MSP 5 cm above the glabella.

OF
- Patient PA erect or prone with MSP centred to the IR in the grid device.
- EAMs equidistant from IR.
- Adjust head until the radiographic baseline and MSP are perpendicular to the IR.
- CR to pass through the MSP at the glabella.

Lateral
- From the erect OF position, turn the patient's head to bring the affected side closer to the IR in the grid device.
- MSP parallel and interpupillary line perpendicular to the IR.
- Centre midway between the glabella and inion (external occipital protruberance), 5 cm superior to the EAM.

Alternative projection

OF 30° cranial (reverse Townes)

- Patient PA erect or prone with MSP centred to the IR in the grid device.
- Forehead and nose in contact with the centre of the grid device.
- EAMs equidistant from IR.
- Adjust head until the radiographic baseline and MSP are perpendicular to the IR.
- Tube angled 30° cranially.
- Centre to the MSP to exit 5 cm above the glabella.

Alternative projection

FO

- Patient AP erect or supine with MSP centred to the IR in the grid device.
- EAMs equidistant from IR.
- Adjust head until the radiographic baseline and MSP are perpendicular to the IR.
- Centre to the MSP at the glabella.

Additional projection

OF 15° caudal

- Patient PA erect or prone with MSP centred to the IR in the grid device.
- Forehead and nose in contact with the centre of the grid device.

- EAMs equidistant from IR.
- Adjust head until the radiographic baseline and MSP are perpendicular to the IR.
- Tube angled 15° caudally.
- Centre to the MSP at the external occipital protuberance to exit at the level of the nasion.

Additional projection

To demonstrate the base of the skull and cranial foramina.

SMV

- Patient supine or erect at least 30 cm away from the IR.
- Hyperextend the neck until the vertex of the skull rests on the grid device.
- MSP perpendicular to and interpupillary line parallel to the plane of the IR.
- Centre to the MSP between the angles of the mandible.

NB: This is a difficult position for the patient to achieve and maintain and may require modification to technique to produce an optimum image.

Additional modality

- CT investigations have largely replaced plain film imaging of the skull.

Small bowel enema

Patient preparation

The patient eats a low-residue diet for 2 days prior to the examination so that the colon is as free from debris as possible.

Basic projections

- The patient's throat is anaesthetised either with a lidocaine spray or by means of a tetracaine lozenge.
- Under fluoroscopic control a tube with a stiff guide wire is introduced transnasally and advanced through the stomach and duodenum until it reaches the duodenojejunal flexure.
- A barium suspension is rapidly introduced under fluoroscopic control and spot films are taken as required until the solution reaches the colon.
- Dependent upon department protocol water may then be introduced via the tube.
- Radiographs of the abdomen in the supine and the prone position are taken as indicated.

Patient aftercare

Nil by mouth for 4–5 hours post procedure.

Alternative modalities

- RNI can be used to measure the gastric emptying rate and in the diagnosis of reflux from the stomach.
- Endoscopy of the colon under fluoroscopic control shows good results in the detection of malignant tumours and larger polyps.
- Positron emission tomography (PET) is useful in tumour staging and in the detection of recurrence of pathology.

Sternoclavicular joint

Both sternoclavicular joints are generally imaged to exclude subluxation or dislocation.

Basic projections

PA

- Patient PA erect with MSP central and perpendicular to the grid device.
- Shoulders in the same transverse plane with arms by the sides.
- CR to pass through the MSP at the sternal notch.
- Exposure on suspended respiration.

Anterior obliques
- From the PA erect position, rotate the patient 45° towards the affected side.
- Horizontal CR at the level of T2–T3 to the sternoclavicular joint nearest the IR.
- Both obliques are generally imaged for comparison.

Sternum

Basic projections

Lateral
- Patient erect with lateral aspect of chest against the grid device.
- MSP parallel to IR.
- Shoulders pulled well back.
- Centre midway between the sternal notch and the xiphisternum.
- Exposure on full inspiration.

LAO (erect)
- From the PA erect position, rotate the patient 45° towards the right. *LEFT*
- Position the right arm above the IR.
- CR to pass midway between the sternal notch and the xiphisternum.
- Exposure on arrested respiration.

NB: A breathing technique can be used to blur the ribs by using a low mA and a long exposure time.

Alternative projection

LAO (prone)

- From the prone position, rotate the patient 45° towards the ~~right~~ LEFT.
- Position the right arm above the head on the pillow.
- Flex the right hip and knee to maintain balance.
- CR to pass midway between the sternal notch and the xiphisternum.
- Exposure on arrested respiration.

NB: This projection is not recommended for trauma cases as the additional information it provides is limited whilst the prone position is difficult for the patient to achieve.

Subtalar joint (see also Ankle)

Basic projection

Medial obliques

- Patient supine/seated with the affected ankle resting on the IR.

- Foot dorsiflexed to avoid superimposition of the calcaneum on the joint space.
- From the AP position the ankle is rotated 45° internally.
- Centre just distal to the lateral malleolus:
  - CR angled 40° cranially to demonstrate the anterior portion of the posterior talocalcaneal articulation
  - CR angled 30° cranially to demonstrate the articulation between the talus and sustentaculum
  - CR angled 10° cranially to demonstrate the posterior portion of the posterior talocalcaneal articulation.

Basic projection

To demonstrate the posterior subtalar joint.

Lateral oblique
- Patient supine/seated with the affected ankle resting on the IR.
- Foot dorsiflexed to avoid superimposition of the calcaneum on the joint space.
- From the AP position the ankle is rotated 45° externally.
- CR angled 15° cranially.
- Centre just distal and anterior to the medial malleolus.

Alternative modality

- MRI is preferred to plain film investigation because of its multiplanar capabilities.

Symphysis menti (see Mandible)

Symphysis pubis (see Pelvis)

Teeth (see Bitewing radiography; Cephalometry; Dental panoramic tomography; Occlusal radiography; Periapical radiography)

Temporomandibular joints (TMJs)

Basic projections

OF 35°

- Patient PA erect or prone with MSP centred to an IR in a grid device.
- Forehead and nose in contact with the centre of the grid device.
- EAMs equidistant from IR.
- Adjust head until the radiographic baseline is perpendicular to the IR.
- Tube angled 35° cranially.
- Centre to the MSP through the TMJs.

Lateral obliques
- From the erect OF position, turn the patient's head to bring the side under investigation closer to the IR in the grid device.
- MSP parallel to and interpupillary line perpendicular to the IR.
- Tube angled 25° caudally.
- Centre 5 cm above EAM, remote from IR. CR should pass through the TMJ nearer the IR.

NB: Images are taken with the mouth open and again with the mouth closed. Care should be taken to label the images correctly.
NB: Both sides are examined for comparison.

Alternative projection

Images of the TMJs with mouth open and closed can also be obtained using a dental panoramic unit with the appropriate settings.

Thoracic inlet

Usually requested to identify soft tissue swellings and/or their effect on the airway.

Basic projections

AP
- Patient erect or supine with MSP central and perpendicular to the grid device.

- Chin raised to bring the radiographic baseline to 20°.
- Centre to the sternal notch.
- Exposure is made while the patient performs the Valsalva manoeuvre.

Lateral
- Patient erect with shoulder of affected side against the grid device.
- MSP parallel to IR.
- Chin raised slightly.
- Shoulders pulled well back to enable visualisation of the trachea.
- Centre at the level of the sternal notch.
- Exposure is made while the patient performs the Valsalva manoeuvre.

NB: The entire length of the trachea can be imaged using a high kVp technique.

Thoracic vertebrae

Basic projections GRID

AP 100cm BROAD 30X40cm

- Patient supine with MSP aligned to the centre of the IR in the grid device.
- Head supported on low pillow or pad.

- Centre three-quarters of the way down from the sternal notch to the xiphisternum.
- Exposure on arrested expiration.

Lateral 100cm Fine focus 30x40cm

- Patient lies in the lateral position with the MSP parallel to the IR.
- The mid-coronal plane is aligned to the centre of the IR in the grid device.
- Arms on the pillow, knees and hips flexed to stabilise.
- Centre at the level of the inferior angle of the scapula, 2.5 cm posterior to the mid-axillary line.
- Exposure on arrested expiration. 115 - 150 FFD

NB: A breathing technique can be used to blur the ribs by using a low mA and a long exposure time. ✳

Thumb

Basic projections
AP 100cm Fine focus 18x24cm

- With patient standing or sitting, adjust body to ensure that thumb, elbow and shoulder are at the same height.

- Extend the affected arm and rotate internally to place the posterior aspect of the thumb in contact with and central to the IR.
- Hyperextend the hand to ensure that the soft tissue of the ulnar aspect does not obscure the first carpometacarpal joint.
- Centre to the first carpometacarpal joint.

Lateral
- Place the affected hand palmar surface down onto IR.
- Thumb abducted.
- Elevate the palmar surface of the hand until the thumb is in the true lateral position.
- Centre to the first carpometacarpal joint.

Alternative projection

If the AP position is impossible for the patient to achieve, the following horizontal beam technique can be employed.

AP
- Patient erect with posterior shoulder of the affected side in contact with vertical IR.
- Displace the IR laterally.
- Flex the elbow, raise the hand to the level of the shoulder and place the dorsal aspect of the thumb on the vertical IR.

- Some lateral rotation of the patient may be required to achieve this position.
- Centre to the first carpometacarpal joint.

Tibia

Basic projections

AP   *100cm   Fine Focus   35×43cm*

- Patient supine/seated with the affected lower limb resting on the IR.
- Dorsiflex foot to avoid superimposition of the calcaneum on the tibiotalar joint space.
- Internally rotate the lower limb to bring the malleoli equidistant from the IR.
- Centre midway between ankle and knee joints.

Lateral   *As above*

- Patient rotated to the affected side with knee flexed and supported on a pad.
- Lower limb resting on the IR with malleoli superimposed.
- Centre midway between ankle and knee joints.

Toes (see also Foot)

Toes may be imaged individually or all together. If the image of a single toe is required, the practice of including other toes to better identify the one under investigation is now in question, as this may contravene IR(ME)R 2000.

Basic projections   18 x 24cn   Fine focus

AP (dorsiplantar) 1st–5th   100 FFD

- Patient supine/sitting with the knees flexed.
- Sole of the affected foot resting on the IR.
- Centre to the base of the 3rd metatarsophalangeal joint (or individual digit).

AP (dorsiplantar) oblique 1st–5th

- From the AP position, rotate the leg medially to raise the lateral aspect of the foot until an angle of 30° is formed between the plantar surface of the foot and the IR.
- Centre to the base of the 3rd metatarsophalangeal joint (or individual digit).

NB: If individual toes are being imaged, centre to the toe under investigation at the metatarsophalangeal joint.

Lateral hallux

- From the AP position, rotate the leg medially until the plantar aspect of the foot is perpendicular to the IR.
- Dorsiflex the hallux or plantarflex the toes not under investigation and immobilise.
- Centre to the PIP joint.

Tomography

Conventional tomography uses the synchronised movement of the tube and IR during an exposure to 'blur' structures above and below a plane of interest, making them invisible on the resultant radiograph. The patient is positioned as usual for a projection, and the height of the organ of interest is carefully set to coincide with the pivot point of the tube motion. This effectively produces a sharp image of the layer at the level of the fulcrum. The thickness of this layer is inversely proportional to the exposure angle. Additional attachments for conventional x-ray equipment allow a linear movement which can acquire tomographic images during, for example, an IVU.

Trachea (see Thoracic inlet)

Ulna (see Forearm)

Ulnar groove (see *also* Elbow;
Olecranon process)

Basic projection

Modified axial
- The elbow and shoulder joints should be in the same horizontal plane.
- Place the fully flexed elbow onto the IR.
- Posterior aspect of humerus in contact with IR.
- Place the palm of the hand facing the shoulder.
- Externally rotate the arm through 45°.
- Centre over the medial epicondyle of the humerus.

Alternative modality

- MRI is the method of choice for investigation of possible ulnar nerve compression.

Urinary tract (see Abdomen; Bladder;
Cystography; Cystourethrography;
Intravenous urography)

Wrist

Basic projections

PA *1000cm fine focus 18x24cm*

- Adjust table height until affected forearm rests on the examination table at shoulder height.
- Flex elbow, place wrist onto IR and slightly flex the fingers.
- Centre midway between the styloid processes.

Lateral *As above*

- From the PA position rotate the forearm externally until the hand is in a lateral position.
- Rotate the wrist another 5° externally to ensure that the styloid processes are superimposed.
- Centre to the radial styloid process.

Zygomatic arch (see *also* Facial bones)

Basic projections

OF axial (modified reverse Townes)
- Patient prone or erect facing IR.
- MSP perpendicular and centred to the IR in the grid device.
- Forehead in contact with the IR.
- EAMs equidistant from the IR.
- Radiographic baseline perpendicular to the IR.
- Tube angled 30° cranially.
- IR displaced appropriately.
- Centre to the MSP to emerge through the zygomatic arches.

NB: A reduction of approximately 10 kVp to the standard Townes exposure is required.

Tangential (modified SMV)
- Patient supine or erect at least 30 cm away from the IR.
- Hyperextend the neck until the vertex of the skull rests on the grid device.
- MSP perpendicular to and interpupillary line parallel to the plane of the IR.

- Centre to the MSP at a point 2.5 cm posterior to the outer canthus of the eye to pass through the zygomatic arches.

NB: A reduction of 10–15 kVp to the standard SMV exposure is required.

Contrast media

CONTRAST MEDIA

X-ray

Different tissue types within the body attenuate the x-ray beam to a degree that is directly related to the thickness, density and atomic number of the element. The result is a variety of absorption coefficients throughout the area under examination which affects the radiographic contrast of the image produced, e.g. from heart muscle in the mediastinum to air in the lungs in chest radiography. Delineation of these two structures will be evident on the image because of the naturally existing contrast.

However, if two organs have similar densities and similar atomic numbers, as in the contents of the abdomen, no natural contrast exists and therefore they will not be individually visualised on a radiograph. A limitation of all plain x-ray examinations is that most of the soft tissue structures of the body are of similar radiographic density. It is therefore necessary to introduce a substance into the body that will increase the radiographic contrast of an area where previously contrast was low or absent. This is achieved by altering the density and the average atomic number of the area under investigation. The development of contrast-enhancing agents has made it possible to visualise an organ, the surface of an organ or the lumen of an organ that would not normally be visible on an x-ray image.

There are numerous types of contrast medium which, dependent upon their physical and chemical properties, are intended for different x-ray examination types. They can be administered orally, rectally, intravenously or subcutaneously. Radiological examinations use contrast media of varying volume, strength and type, dependent upon the examination, the patient profile and radiologist's preference.

Desirable features of contrast media are numerous, the most important being to ensure that they are not detrimental to patient well-being. They should cause negligible distress to the patient on introduction, no adverse reactions post introduction and no permanent alteration to the organ they target. They must be easy to administer and remain stable within the body so as not to dissociate into toxic ions. Once in the body they need to concentrate in the intended area and remain unchanged by, for example, organ contents, in order to allow that organ to be accurately demonstrated. Viscosity of the contrast medium on introduction is significant to both patient comfort and the success of the procedure being carried out. Elimination should be rapid. Cost should not be prohibitive to their use.

The contrast media traditionally used in radiology departments can be divided into two main groups: positive and negative contrast media. They are either insoluble or water-soluble (the latter clearing easily from virtually any body cavity). The water-soluble contrast media represent the largest group of iodinated contrast media. They do not cross either the intact gastrointestinal tract (GIT) mucosa or blood–brain barrier.

Positive contrast media

These are either barium or iodine based and radiopaque as a result of their ability to attenuate the x-ray beam. Positive contrast media increase the atomic number of the areas they are being used to demonstrate relative to the surrounding tissue. The contrast medium absorbs the x-rays and the organ under investigation appears radiopaque on the resultant radiograph.

Barium

This is used in the form of barium sulphate, a suspension of insoluble particles, almost exclusively for the GIT, passing through it without dissociating into ions. It is administered orally or rectally during fluoroscopy or to enhance CT images of the abdomen and pelvis.

Advantages   Coming in various forms from the manufacturers, it is available ready-made in cans, as a powder to which water is added, as aerated liquid preparations and ready-prepared in plastic bags for specific examinations. A relatively inexpensive medium, it has excellent coating properties with flexibility of use as a result of the differing concentrations available, dependent on its dilution with water, for the region of the GIT under examination. Double-contrast examinations of the GIT use air or carbon dioxide as the second contrast medium. For the upper GIT this is generally in the form of gas-forming granules and room air is used for the lower tract. A double-contrast study gives optimal mucosal detail and avoids small anomalies being concealed by large volumes of positive contrast media.

Disadvantages   One practical disadvantage of using barium sulphate is that subsequent examinations may be difficult as once in the intestinal tract it takes time to clear.

Precautions   Adequate hydration of the patient post procedure is recommended.

Contraindications   If a perforation of the bowel is suspected the use of barium sulphate is contraindicated as its presence in the GIT can cause, along with pain and shock, a chemical peritonitis which can prove to be fatal in extreme cases. In these circumstances or where there is a suspected sinus or fistula, water-soluble contrast media should be used. The same applies in the upper GIT should a perforated ulcer be suspected.

Iodine

Iodine-based contrast agents are the largest group used in medical imaging. Although there are other elements with higher atomic numbers, iodine is suitable as a radiographic contrast medium because it is the only one with chemical characteristics that allow it to develop into soluble compounds that have low toxicity. There are numerous brands on the market with each one prepared for specific use(s) and for the most they are used intravenously. The exception is Gastrografin, a water-soluble iodinated contrast medium for oral administration.

Precautions The rate of adverse reactions to intravascular iodinated contrast media is relatively low but certain patient groups show a greater predisposition. The Royal College of Radiologists[6,7] has identified those they consider to be at a higher risk of having adverse reactions. These high-risk patients include those:

- with previous severe reaction to contrast medium
- with asthma or significant allergic history
- with proven or suspected sensitivity to iodine
- on beta-blockers
- with heart disease
- who are infants or small children
- with hepatic failure
- with moderate or severe renal function impairment
- with diabetes mellitus
- with multiple myeloma
- who are poorly hydrated
- with sickle cell anaemia

- with thyrotoxicosis as a result of high iodine loading
- who are pregnant.

Negative contrast media

These are radiolucent with low attenuation of the x-ray beam. They have low atomic weights and include air, carbon dioxide (CO_2) and xenon.

Air

Air is generally used in double-contrast examinations which include arthrography and investigations of the GIT. In the lower GIT the colon is first filled with barium, the barium is then drained out, leaving just a thin layer of the material on the lining of the large intestine. Air is then introduced into the large intestine via the rectum.

Advantages	This technique provides a more detailed picture of the lining of the colon, improving the procedure's ability to detect small polyps or inflammation.
Disadvantages	The addition of air into a region, e.g. joint space or

internal organ, can cause discomfort to the patient as it can take a few days for it to be absorbed by the body tissues.

CO_2

The most common use of CO_2 is in diagnostic vascular imaging and vascular interventions in both the arterial and venous circulation of patients who are not suitable candidates for iodinated contrast media.

Advantages   As it is a normal constituent of the body the possibility of allergic reaction is eliminated, thus making it a possible alternative in patients with a history of adverse reaction to iodinated contrast media.

It is easily eliminated and will not cause any renal toxicity so can be safely used in patients in renal failure. In addition, it is not hyperosmolar so it is not seen to be dangerous for most cardiac patients.

Disadvantages	As it is less dense than iodinated contrast media, CO_2 will produce images of a slightly inferior image quality.
Contraindications	It should never be used in the coronary and cerebral circulatory systems as there is the risk of a gas embolism.

Xenon

The inhalation of xenon gas is used in a highly specialised form of lung or brain imaging. These CT techniques are only available in a very few locations worldwide.

MRI

MRI contrast media work to change the signal intensity between tissue containing the contrast medium and tissue that does not, so increasing the contrast on the resultant image. The volume and concentration of contrast media used in MRI tend to be less than that used in traditional radiological procedures. MRI contrast media can be organ specific or have a more general use for various tissue types.

Gadolinium (Gd)

This heavy metal is contained in most MRI contrast media and appears to have an excellent safety profile. Adverse reactions do occur but appear to be less common than reactions to traditional iodinated contrast media and are comparable with non-iodinated contrast media. They tend to be unrelated to the dose given and tolerable by patients in some increased risk groups.

The most common reactions include injection site pain, fever, headache, itching, skin flushing, watery eyes and nausea. Less common reactions include abdominal discomfort or pain, agitation, diarrhoea, joint pain, muscle pain or spasm, nosebleeds, pain or swelling of eye, tinnitus and facial oedema. Severe anaphylactic reactions are rare with a low reported mortality rate.

Ultrasound

Ultrasound contrast media work by increasing the reflection and refraction of the ultrasonic waves. Intravenous vascular-enhancing contrast agents in the form of stabilised microbubbles of air are highly echogenic, small enough to pass capillary beds and remain in the bloodstream long enough to be clinically useful. They are excellent reflectors of ultrasound waves with little risk of adverse reaction to the patient.

There are a growing number of contrast media being developed for use with ultrasound and application for their use is growing in tandem with their development. Contrast techniques are used in procedures which include cardiac and vascular ultrasound, echocardiology, the evaluation of fallopian tube patency in patients with fertility problems and vesicoureteral reflux in children. These procedures are of benefit to the patient as they carry no radiation burden.

Recommendations for best practice

Adverse reactions fall into two categories. The first is influenced by the chemical and physical properties of the contrast medium which are believed to interfere with the homeostasis of the body, especially the blood and the circulatory system. Iodine concentration, volume of contrast medium injected and rate of injection also play a part in the reaction process. The second category is idiosyncratic, unaffected by the elements in the first category, and in presentation resemble an allergic/anaphylactic reaction.

The points noted below may provide a better understanding of the aetiology of possible adverse reactions.

- A thorough knowledge of patient history should be ascertained before the injection of any contrast medium to identify any patient who may fall into a high-risk group.
- The weight of children should be known prior to any procedure involving the use of a contrast medium in order to ensure that the correct dosage is administered.
- The contrast medium to be used should be checked to ensure that it is the correct type and within its expiry date. The quantity and concentration to be used should be verified as appropriate for the procedure being carried out. The contrast agent should be clear and the condition of its glass container should show no hint of contamination.

- Records should be kept identifying the name of the person who administered the contrast medium, the date of administration, the type, quantity and concentration of the contrast agent, plus any adverse reaction, no matter how mild, that the patient experienced. In addition, it is recommended that the expiry date and the batch number of the contrast medium are noted.

- It should also be remembered that it is essential to have a request form signed by an appropriate medical practitioner.
- Precautions should be taken to ensure patient and staff safety. Techniques should be employed to remove the possibility of cross-infection for the patient and needlestick injuries for the person administering the contrast medium. Waste disposal protocols should be adhered to.
- It is important that procedures are put in place to allow any adverse reaction that occurs in the x-ray department to be dealt with swiftly so that a favourable outcome for the patient is achieved. All staff should be acquainted with the departmental protocols regarding adverse reactions to contrast media. Oxygen should be available in every room where contrast media are

used. The radiographer has a responsibility to ensure that there is an appropriately stocked emergency drugs cabinet at hand along with an emergency trolley equipped to provide resuscitation and monitoring equipment. All staff in attendance at procedures involving contrast media should be trained in cardiopulmonary resuscitation and be familiar with the local code to call the 'crash team' in cases of severe reactions. Close observation of the patient before, during and after the administration of a contrast medium can often alert the radiographer to any change in patient condition. When intravascular contrast has been introduced the needle/Venflon used should remain in situ for at least 5 minutes post injection to allow rapid access for the administration of remedial drug therapy should it be required. The patient should never be left alone after the administration of a contrast medium as adverse reaction is unpredictable and patient condition can change rapidly. The most severe reactions tend to occur within 20 minutes of administration of an intravenous contrast medium so the patient should be monitored for at least this length of time.

Chemical and physical properties of contrast media

Iodinated contrast media can be classified into two groups: high-osmolar (HOCM), also known as ionic contrast media, and low-osmolar (LOCM), or non-ionic contrast media.

A primary difference between ionic and non-ionic contrast media is that an ionic (HOCM) compound dissociates into charged particles when it enters a solution such as blood. Ionic contrast media break down into positively charged cations and negatively charged anions. For every three iodine molecules present in an ionic contrast solution, one cation and one anion form. Ionic contrast media are therefore referred to as 3 : 2 compounds. This dissociation of molecules is responsible for the increased osmolality in blood. The osmolality of a solution measures the number of dissolved molecules and particles in a defined unit of a solution and is expressed in milliosmoles per kilogram (mOsmol/kg).

Human blood plasma has an osmolality of 300 mOsmol/kg; ionic contrast has a value of 1300–2000 mOsmol/kg. This is significant as the osmolality of the contrast medium is 5 times higher than that of blood plasma so is said to be hypertonic. It is this hypertonicity to which the toxicity of contrast media is generally attributed.

The charged ions formed as a result of the dissociation in ionic contrast media have the potential to disrupt electrical charges associated with the heart and the brain. For this reason they should not be used in the subarachnoid space. The sensations of heat, discomfort and pain on introduction of a contrast medium experienced by some patients have been attributed to the osmolality of the contrast being injected.

Non-ionic media on the other hand do not disassociate on entering a solution. For every three iodine molecules present in a non-ionic solution, one neutral molecule is produced. Non-ionic contrast media are therefore referred to as 3 : 1 compounds. The osmolality of non-ionic contrast media is in the region of 500–800 mOsmol/kg and although this is approximately half the osmolality for the same iodine content as ionic media, it is still hypertonic when compared with blood. The closer the osmolality of a contrast medium to that of blood, the better the tolerance of its presence within the body and the less likelihood there is of an adverse reaction.

A non-ionic medium therefore appears to be the contrast medium that is least likely to cause adverse reaction on administration. Cost, however, is up to 10 times more than for an ionic contrast medium so selective use may be necessary as finance could be prohibitive to its continual use.

Iodine concentration and viscosity

The iodine concentration of a contrast agent is determined by the number of milligrams of iodine molecules in a millilitre (mg/ml) of a solution. The higher the concentration of iodine, the greater the absorption of x-ray photons and therefore the contrast medium will be more radiopaque. However, the risk of adverse reaction is increased with contrast media containing higher iodine concentrations. If large amounts of contrast are required for an examination it is advisable to use those with a lower concentration.

The iodine content of the contrast medium is related to its viscosity. The higher the concentration, the greater the viscosity and therefore the greater the pressure required to inject it. It is this 'thickness' that causes resistance to its flow through a needle or catheter. The length and diameter of the introducing tube/needle being used add to this resistance and further limit the rate at which contrast can be injected.

A very viscous contrast medium will be slow to inject and as a result may lead to inadequate visualisation of a vessel, e.g. during an arteriogram. Reducing the concentration will reduce the viscosity but this may result in inadequate opacification of the ROI. Viscosity is reduced when the contrast medium is warmed to approximately body temperature, so reducing the impedance to flow.

Both osmolality and viscosity are directly related to the concentration of the contrast medium. The ability of a contrast medium to opacify rises with its increasing concentration. Viscosity and osmolality also increase in line with any rise in concentration and, as is known, add to the chance of adverse reaction. This being so, most contrast agents are available in a number of different concentrations.

Volume and rate of injection

The rate at which a contrast medium is injected affects the likelihood of reaction. The faster contrast is injected, the greater the risk of adverse reaction. When a contrast medium is injected into the vascular system there is an increase in the number of particles present within it. The contrast medium's particles draw plasma water to them so water from the cells moves into the vascular system via the capillary membrane to equalise the situation. As a result of increased fluid volume, the vessels dilate in an attempt to compensate for the increased fluid volume. This mechanism cannot always deal with the volume of fluid present, especially when a large volume of contrast is being injected rapidly, and this can result in fluid extravasation into the surrounding tissue. This in itself can cause a patient great discomfort. Abnormal increases in the volume of circulating fluids or blood (hypervolaemia) and rapid movement of fluid through the vascular system is thought to be a factor contributing to pain linked with vessel dilation, nausea, vomiting, flushing, damage to the vascular endothelium and dehydration. This osmotic effect has the ability to cause expansion of the renal arteries, so releasing vasoconstrictors. This leads to rapid opening and closing of the arteries which culminates in a reduced blood supply to the kidneys, leading to total kidney failure in extreme cases.

Predisposing factors for this include known renal function impairment, diabetes mellitus, dehydration, age, multiple myeloma, large dosage and the use of other nephrotoxic drugs. To minimise the risk of this contrast-induced nephropathy in patients with a known predisposing condition, non-ionic contrast media should be used with as low a dose as is possible to provide the maximum amount of diagnostic information. Dehydration is not recommended and at least 2 days should be left between examinations requiring contrast media.

In an attempt to regulate fluid overload in the vascular system where the kidneys are non-functional, the fluid seeks alternative routes of elimination. This will result in fluid overload in other body systems with one major effect of this being pulmonary oedema.

Idiosyncratic reactions

This type of reaction resembles an allergic/anaphylactic reaction with antibodies forming in response to the symptoms of an allergy. The resultant antibody–antigen response stimulates the release of naturally occurring histamine. Histamine acts to constrict smooth muscle, increase heart rate, decrease blood pressure, dilate arterioles, constrict venules, produce localised oedema and increase gastric and mucous secretions. Primarily, histamine will have an effect on the cardiovascular, gastrointestinal, respiratory and central nervous systems. The release of histamine as a response to an anaphylactic reaction can lead to the vascular system becoming overloaded and so histamine extravasates into surrounding tissues. This results in reddening, inflammation and possibly localised swelling.

Idiosyncratic reactions vary in degree, are numerous and are classed as minor, moderate or severe. This classification reflects the type of treatment required to treat the adverse reaction.

- *Minor reactions* include flushing, metallic taste in the mouth, urticaria, sneezing, nausea, vomiting, a mild rash and arm pain or a tingling sensation. Related to dose and speed of injection, the risk of these occurrences is reduced if LOCM is used. Slow introduction of the contrast will decrease the occurrence of headaches and metallic taste. These reactions require no treatment other than reassurance of the patient.

• *Moderate reactions*, occurring less frequently, include more severe urticaria, hypotension, bronchospasm and facial oedema. Dependent upon patient profile it may be advantageous to treat with prophylactic steroids prior to contrast medium injection. The use of non-ionic contrast media is again recommended to reduce the risk.

• *Severe reactions* occur very rarely and require immediate treatment. These reactions include hypotensive shock, convulsions, and respiratory and cardiac arrest. Occasionally they can prove to be fatal. Appropriate rapid treatment is required.

SECTION 4

Radiological examination of women of reproductive capacity

Radiological investigations of the abdominal and pelvic areas in the case of pregnancy are contraindicated and a system is required to eliminate this possibility. Women in the very early stages may not even be aware that they are pregnant and therefore merely asking them to confirm that they are not pregnant is unreliable. A more accurate method is to establish the first day of the onset of the last menstrual period and record this on the request card. The patient should sign to affirm that the date has been recorded correctly. Individual reproductive status can then be calculated and a form of risk assessment used to determine the benefit/risk of proceeding with the examination based on local guidelines and further discussion with the patient.

Appointments for non-urgent radiological examinations of the abdomen, lumbar spine, pelvis, hips, barium examinations, urinary tract investigations and CT scans on women of reproductive capacity can be arranged to coincide with the first few days of the next menstrual period. Urgent examinations outwith the local guidelines are undertaken at the discretion of the referring clinician or radiologist singly or jointly, with a signature to take responsibility. A more detailed discussion of possible pregnancy can be undertaken at this stage and/or a pregnancy test used for better confirmation. The patient should be made aware of any potential risks to a fetus.

The National Radiological Protection Board (NRPB) recommends that while conventional diagnostic procedures carry no substantial risk to the early conceptus, the use of high-dose procedures should be avoided, e.g. those entailing tens of mGy such as a barium enema examination or a CT investigation of the abdomen and/or pelvis. In practice, this means the use of a 28-day rule for general procedures and a 10-day rule for higher dose investigations.

The possible effects of irradiating a fetus

Teratogenesis

It has been established from animal studies that irradiation when an organ is being formed can damage that organ, and a human fetus is therefore at risk from weeks 2 to 25 after conception. Evidence from atomic bomb survivors shows that detriment may be expressed as malformation of specific organs and/or mental retardation, dependent on the stage of gestation when irradiation occurs. During the first trimester there are a large number of stem cells in the embryo which are very radiosensitive and susceptible to death or damage. At the preimplantation stage no malformations are expressed although embryonic death occurs if exposed to doses between 50 and 150 mGy. At the organogenesis stage congenital malformations may include growth inhibition, microcephaly, mental retardation, damage to sense organs, genital deformities, etc. Some of these deformities may be fatal and cause neonatal death. Most skeletal damage occurs between weeks 3 and 20 of gestation.

Genetic injury

There is a measurable risk of sterility or serious genetic injury occurring within the first two generations following high-dose irradiation of the fetus. Animal studies suggest that germ cells are more sensitive during meiotic divisions, which occur during the last trimester of pregnancy in the human.

Cancer production

Some studies have shown a relationship between childhood cancer and irradiation in utero. The United Nations Scientific Committee on the Effects of Atomic Radiation (UNSCEAR) assessed the increased fatal cancer risk from radiation to the fetus to be approximately twice the risk of cancer in an adult. The gestational age at irradiation appears to be less relevant in these cases, e.g. leukaemia can be induced at any stage of development in utero, although it occurs more often if the fetus is exposed in the first trimester. The NRPB has also estimated that fetal exposure to high-dose diagnostic radiological examinations in the early gestational stages may result in a doubling of the incidence of fatal childhood cancer compared with an unexposed population.

SECTION

4

SECTION 5

Appendices

Dose reference levels

The NRPB has compiled a database of radiation doses received by patients during the most common diagnostic investigations in order to provide national reference levels. The use of local diagnostic reference levels (DRLs) to monitor patient safety is an employer's responsibility under IR(ME)R 2000. These quote effective doses, measured in mSv, which are used to predict the risk of harm from radiation to a patient. However, the effective dose is a derived unit and not easily used in clinical practice. The table below shows some DRLs for entrance surface dose (mGy) which is the unit measured by thermoluminescent dosimeters (TLDs).

Diagnostic reference levels for some common radiographic examinations

Radiograph	Entrance surface dose (mGy)
Chest PA	0.2
Chest lateral	1.0
Skull lateral	1.5
Skull AP/PA	3.0
Thoracic vertebrae AP	3.5
Pelvis AP	4.0
Abdomen AP	6.0
Lumbar vertebrae AP	6.0
Thoracic vertebrae lateral	10.0
Lumbar vertebrae lateral	14.0
Lumbosacral junction	26.0

Abbreviations

?	Query
#	Fracture
<	less than
>	more than
↑	raised/hyper
↓	lowered/hypo
2°	secondary deposits
AAA	abdominal aortic aneurysm
Ab	abortion
AC	acromioclavicular
ACL	anterior cruciate ligament
ADH	antidiuretic hormone
ADR	adverse drug reaction
AE	after evacuation
AF	atrial fibrillation
Ag	antigen
AIDS	acquired immune deficiency syndrome
AIS	adolescent idiopathic scoliosis
ALARA	as low as reasonably achievable
ALARP	as low as reasonably practicable
ALD	alcoholic liver disease
AM	after micturition
AML	acute myeloid leukaemia
AP	anteroposterior
ARDS	acute respiratory distress syndrome

ARF	acute renal failure
ASD	atrial septal defect
ASIS	anterior superior iliac spine
ATN	acute tubular necrosis
AVB	atrioventricular block
AVF	arteriovenous fistula
AVH	acute viral hepatitis
AVR	aortic valve replacement
AXR	abdominal x-ray
Ba	barium
BaSO₄	barium sulphate
BE	barium enema
BI	bony injury
BIR	British Institute of Radiologists
BMI	body mass index
BMR	basal metabolic rate
BMT	bone marrow transplant
BMUS	British Medical Ultrasound Society
BP	blood pressure
BPD	biparietal diameter
BPI	blood pressure index
bpm	beats per minute
BSR	blood sedimentation rate
C	cervical vertebrae
Ca	carcinoma
CABG	coronary artery bypass graft
CAD	coronary artery disease

CAPD	continuous ambulatory peritoneal dialysis
CBD	common bile duct
CBF	cerebral blood flow
CBP	chronic back pain
cc	cubic centimetre
CC	craniocaudal
CCF	congestive cardiac failure
CCU	coronary care unit
CDH	congenital dysplasia of the hip
CF	cystic fibrosis
CHD	coronary heart disease
CHF	congestive heart failure
CML	chronic myeloid leukaemia
CNS	central nervous system
C/O	complains of
COAD	chronic obstructive airway disease
COPD	chronic obstructive pulmonary disease
CoR	College of Radiographers
COSHH	Control of Substances Hazardous to Health
CP	cerebral palsy
CPB	cardiopulmonary bypass
CR	central ray
CSF	cerebrospinal fluid
CT	computed tomography

CVA	cerebrovascular accident
CVP	central venous pressure
CXR	chest x-ray
D	absorbed dose
D&C	dilatation and curettage
DDH	developmental dysplasia of the hip
DE	dose equivalent
DEXA	dual energy x-ray absorptiometry
DIB	difficulty in breathing
DIP	distal interphalangeal joint
DM	diabetes mellitus
DNA	deoxyribonucleic acid; did not attend
DOA	dead on arrival
DRL	diagnostic reference level
DU	duodenal ulcer
DVT	deep vein thrombosis
DXRT	deep x-ray therapy
E	effective dose
EAM	external auditory meatus
ECG	electrocardiogram
EDD	expected delivery date
EEG	electroencephalogram
EMG	electromyogram
ENT	ear, nose and throat
EOP	external occipital protuberance

Ep	epilepsy
ERCP	endoscopic retrograde cholangiopancreatography
ESR	erythrocyte sedimentation rate
ESRF	end stage renal failure
ETT	endotracheal tube
EUA	examination under anaesthetic
FB	foreign body
FDD	focus to detector distance
FDE	fetal dose estimate
FFD	fixed flexion deformity
FH	family history
FHR	fetal heart rate
FID	focus to image distance
FNA	fine needle aspiration
FO	fronto-occipital
FT	follow through (small bowel)
GA	general anaesthetic
GHIF	growth hormone inhibiting factor
GHRF	growth hormone releasing factor
GIT	gastrointestinal tract
GOR	gastro-oesophageal reflux
GU	gastric ulcer; genitourinary
Gy	gray
H_2O	water
Hb	haemoglobin
HDU	high dependency unit

H_E	effective dose equivalent
HGH	human growth hormone
HI	head injury
HIDA	hepatobiliary iminodiacetic acid (scan)
HIV	human immunodeficiency virus
HPC	history of present condition
HRT	hormone replacement therapy
HT	hypertension
H_T	equivalent dose
HVL	half-value layer
IAM	internal auditory meatus
IBD	inflammatory bowel disease
IBS	irritable bowel syndrome
ICP	intracranial pressure
ICRP	International Commission on Radiological Protection
ICU	intensive care unit
IF	internal fixation
IOFB	intraocular foreign body
IOP	intraocular pressure
IPH	intrapartum haemorrhage
IR	image receptor
IR(ME)R	Ionising Radiation (Medical Exposure) Regulations
ITU	intensive therapy unit
IUCD	intrauterine contraceptive device

IUD	intrauterine death
IV	intervertebral; intravenous
IVC	inferior vena cava
IVP	intravenous pyelogram
IVU	intravenous urogram
JCA	juvenile chronic arthritis
JHO	junior house officer
JIS	juvenile idiopathic scoliosis
KUB	kidneys, ureters and bladder
kVp	kilovoltage peak
L	lumbar vertebrae
LA	local anaesthetic
LAO	left anterior oblique
LAT	lateral
LBP	low back pain
LCM	lower costal margin
LFT	liver function test
LIF	left iliac fossa
LLL	left lower lobe
LMP	last menstrual period
LPO	left posterior oblique
LUL	left upper lobe
LV	left ventricle
LVF	left ventricular failure
mA	milliamperes
MABP	mean arterial blood pressure
mAs	milliampere seconds
MC	metacarpal

MCP	metacarpophalangeal
MeV	million electron volts
MI	myocardial infarction
mm	millimetres
MPAP	mean pulmonary artery pressure
MR	magnetic resonance; mitral regurgitation
MRCP	magnetic resonance cholangiopancreatography
MRI	magnetic resonance imaging
MRSA	methicillin-resistant *Staphylococcus aureus*
MS	mitral stenosis; multiple sclerosis
MSP	mid-sagittal plane
MSU	mid-stream urine
mSv	millisieverts
MT	metatarsal
MTP	metatarsophalangeal
MVD	mitral valve disease
Mx	mastectomy
NAD	no abnormality detected/demonstrated
NAI	non-accidental injury
NB	*note bene* (take note)
NBI	no bony injury
NBM	nil by mouth

NCRP	National Commission on Radiological Protection
NFS	no fracture shown
NG	nasogastric; new growth (neoplasm)
NITU	neonatal intensive therapy unit
NM	nuclear medicine
NMR	nuclear magnetic resonance
NND	neonatal death
NPU	not passed urine
NRPB	National Radiological Protection Board
NSAID	non-steroidal anti-inflammatory drug
NWB	non-weight bearing
O_2	oxygen
OA	osteoarthritis
OC	oral contraceptive
OD	overdose
OE	on examination
OF	occipitofrontal
OID	object to image distance
OM	occipitomental
OR	open reduction
ORIF	open reduction internal fixation
OT	occupational therapist
PA	pernicious anaemia; posteroanterior

SECTION
5

PCL	posterior cruciate ligament
PE	pulmonary embolus
PET	positron emission tomography
pH	level of acidity
PID	pelvic inflammatory disease; prolapsed intervertebral disc
PIH	pregnancy-induced hypertension
PIP	proximal interphalangeal
PM	post micturition; post mortem
PNS	post-nasal space
PoP	plaster of Paris
PP	proximal phalanx
PR	per rectum
PSIS	posterior superior iliac spine
PTB	pulmonary tuberculosis
PTC	percutaneous transhepatic cholangiogram
PU	passed urine; peptic ulcer
PUO	pyrexia of unknown origin
PV	per vaginum
Q	radiation quality factor
qv	quod vide (please see)
R	roentgen
RA	rheumatoid arthritis; right auricle (atrium)
Rad	radiation absorbed dose
RAO	right anterior oblique

RAS	renal artery stenosis
RB	recurrent bleed
RCR	Royal College of Radiologists
RDS	respiratory distress syndrome
rem	Roentgen equivalent man
RHD	rheumatic heart disease
RIF	right iliac fossa
RLL	right lower lobe
RNI	radionuclide imaging
ROI	region of interest
RPO	right posterior oblique
RSO	radiation safety officer
RTA	road traffic accident
RUL	right upper lobe
RV	right ventricle
S	sacral vertebrae
SAH	subarachnoid haemorrhage
SCBU	special care baby unit
SDH	subdural haemorrhage
S_E	collective effective dose
SHO	senior house officer
SI	sacroiliac
SID	source to image distance
SIDS	sudden infant death syndrome (cot death)
SIJ	sacroiliac joint
SMV	submentovertical
SOB	shortness of breath

SECTION
5

SOL	space occupying lesion
SoR	Society of Radiographers
SPECT	single photon emission computed tomography
SSD	source to skin distance
STD	sexually transmitted disease
Sv	sievert
SVC	superior vena cava
SXR	skull x-ray
T	thoracic vertebrae
T1	longitudinal magnetisation relaxation time
T2	transverse magnetisation relaxation time
T21	trisomy 21 (Down syndrome)
TAUS	transabdominal ultrasound
TB	tuberculosis
TBI	total body irradiation
THR	total hip replacement
TKR	total knee replacement
TLD	thermoluminescent dosimeter
TMJ	temporomandibular joint
TOF	tracheo-oesophageal fistula
TP	terminal phalanx
TPR	temperature, pulse, respiration
TRUS	transrectal ultrasound
TSS	toxic shock syndrome

TURP	transurethral resection of prostate
TVUS	transvaginal ultrasound
Tx	transplant
UNSCEAR	United Nations Scientific Committee on the Effects of Atomic Radiation
URTI	upper respiratory tract infection
US	ultrasound
UTI	urinary tract infection
VLBW	very low birth weight
V/Q	ventilation/perfusion ratio
VSD	ventricular septal defect
WB	weight bearing
WBC	white blood cell
W_T	tissue weighting factor

Word root

Prefix	Definition	Suffix
a	without; absence of	
ab	from; away from	
abdomin	abdomen	
	pertaining to	ac
acanth	thorny, spiny	
acetabul	acetabulum (hip socket)	
acou	hearing	
acr	extremities; height	
actin	ray; radius	
ad	to; toward	
aden	gland	
adenoid	adenoids	
adren	adrenal gland	
adrenal	adrenal gland	
	of the blood	aemia
aer	air; gas	
	excessive pain	agra
	pertaining to	al
albumin	albumin	
algesi	pain	
	pain	algia
alveol	alveolus	
ambly	dull; dim	
amni	amnion	
amnion	amnion	

Prefix	Definition	Suffix
amyl	starch	
an	without; absence of	
ana	up; again; backward	
andr	male	
angio	vessel	
anis	unequal; dissimilar	
ankyl	crooked; stiff; bent	
ante	before	
anti	against	
antr	antrum	
anu	anus	
aort	aorta	
	removal	*apheresis*
apo	upon	
aponeur	aponeurosis	
appendic	appendix	
	pertaining to	*ar*
arachno	spider-like	
arche	first; beginning	
arteri	artery	
arteriol	arteriole (small artery)	
arthr	joint	
articul	joint	
	pertaining to	*ary*
	enzyme	*ase*
	weakness	*asthenia*
atel	imperfect; incomplete	

APPENDICES

Prefix	Definition	Suffix
ather	yellowish; fatty plaque	
	absence of normal body-opening; occlusion; closure	atresia
atri	atrium	
aur	ear	
aut	self	
axill	armpit	
azot	urea; nitrogen	
bacteri	bacteria	
balan	glans penis	
bi	two	
bil	bile	
bin	two	
blast	developing cell	
blephar	eyelid	
brachi	arm	
brady	slow	
bronch	bronchus	
bronchiol	bronchiole	
bucc	cheek	
burs	bursa (cavity)	
calc	calcium	
cancer	cancer	
	carbon dioxide	capnia
carcin	cancer	
cardi	heart	
carp	carpals	

Prefix	Definition	Suffix
cata	down	
caud	tail; toward the lower part of the body	
cec	caecum	
	hernia; protrusion	*cele*
celi	abdomen	
	surgical puncture to aspirate fluid	*centesis*
ceph	head	
cerebell	cerebellum	
cerebr	cerebrum, brain	
cerumin	cerumen (earwax)	
cervic	cervix	
cheil	lip	
chir	hand	
chol	gall; bile	
cholangi	bile duct	
choledoch	common bile duct	
chondr	cartilage	
chori	chorion	
chrom	colour	
	killing	*cidal*
	break	*clasia*
	break	*clasis*
	break	*clast*
clavic	clavicle	

Prefix	Definition	Suffix
clavicul	clavicle	
	irrigating; washing	clysis
	plural of coccus	cocci
	berry-shaped (form of bacterium)	coccus
col	colon	
colp	vagina	
con	together	
coni	dust	
conjunctiv	conjunctiva	
contra	against	
cor	pupil	
core	pupil	
corne	cornea	
coron	heart	
cortic	cortex	
cost	rib	
crani	cranium	
	separate; secrete	crine
	to separate	crit
cry	cold	
crypt	hidden	
culd	cul-de-sac	
cutane	skin	
cyan	blue	
cyes	pregnancy	
cyst	bladder; sac	

Prefix	Definition	Suffix
	cell	*cyte*
cyto	cell	
dacry	tear; tear duct	
dactyl	fingers or toes	
de	from; down from; lack of	
dent	tooth	
derm	skin	
derma	skin	
	surgical fixation; fusion	*desis*
dextr	right	
dia	complete; thorough	
diaphor	sweat	
diaphragmat	diaphragm	
dipl	two; double	
dips	thirst	
dis	to undo; free from	
disc	intervertebral disc	
distal	furthest away from the centre	
diverticul	diverticulum	
dors	back (of the body)	
	run; running	*drome*
duoden	duodenum	
dur	hard; dura mater	
dynam	power; strength	
dys	difficult; laboured; painful; abnormal	
	pertaining to	*eal*

Prefix	Definition	Suffix
ech	sound	
	stretching out; dilation; expansion	ectasis
ecto	outside; outer	
	excision; surgical removal	ectomy
ectop	located away from usual place	
	displacement	ectopia
electr	electricity; electrical activity	
	swelling	ema
embry	embryo; to be full	
	vomiting	emesis
	blood condition	emia
emmetr	a normal measure	
encephal	brain	
endo	within	
endocrin	endocrine	
enter	intestines	
epi	on; upon; over	
epididym	epididymis	
epiglott	epiglottis	
episi	vulva	
epitheli	epithelium	
	one who	er
erythr	red	
erythro	red	
	condition	esis
eso	inward	

Prefix	Definition	Suffix
esophag	oesophagus	
esthesi	sensation; sensitivity; feeling	
eti	cause (of disease)	
eu	normal; good	
ex	outside; outward	
exo	outside; outward	
extra	outside of; beyond	
faci	face	
femor	femur	
fet	fetus	
	to carry	*fferent*
fibr	fibrous tissue	
fibul	fibula	
gangli	ganglion	
gastro	stomach	
	agent/substance that causes	*gen*
	origin; cause	*genesis*
	producing; originating; causing	*genic*
ger	old age; aged	
geront	old age; aged	
gingiv	gum	
	protein	*globin*
glomerul	glomerulus	
gloss	tongue	
gluc	sweetness; sugar	
glyc	sugar	
glycos	sugar	
gnath	jaw	

SECTION

5

APPENDICES

Prefix	Definition	Suffix
gnos	knowledge	
gon	seed	
	record; x-ray IR	*gram*
	instrument used to record	*graph*
	process of recording	*graphy*
gravid	pregnancy	
gyn	woman	
gynae	woman	
haem	blood	
haemat	blood	
hemi	half	
hepat	liver	
herni	hernia	
heter	other	
hidr	sweat	
hist	tissue	
hom	same	
home	sameness; unchanging	
humer	humerus	
hydr	water	
hymen	hymen	
hyper	above; excessive	
hypn	sleep	
hypo	below; incomplete; deficient	
hyster	uterus	
	diseased; abnormal state	*ia*
	pertaining to	*ial*
	condition; tendency to form	*iasis*

Prefix	Definition	Suffix
iatr	medicine; physician	
	treatment; physician	*iatry*
	pertaining to	*ic*
ichthy	fish	
	one who	*ician*
	seizure; attack	*ictal*
ile	ileum	
ili	ilium	
immun	immune	
in	in; into; not	
infra	under; below	
inter	between	
intra	within	
iri	iris	
irid	iris	
is	equal; same	
isch	deficiency; blockage	
ischi	ischium	
	condition	*ism*
	inflammation	*itis*
jejun	jejunum	
juxta	adjacent to	
kal	potassium	
kary	nucleus	
kerat	cornea; horny tissue; hard	
kin	movement	
kinesi	movement; motion	

Prefix	Definition	Suffix
kyph	hump	
labi	lips	
labyrinth	labyrinth	
lacrim	tear duct; tear	
lact	milk	
lamin	lamina (thin flat plate or layer)	
lapar	abdomen	
laryng	larynx	
later	side	
lei	smooth	
	seizure	*lepsy*
leuk	white	
lingu	tongue	
lip	fat	
lith	stone; calculus	*lith*
lob	lobe	
lord	bent forward	
lymph	lymph	
	loosening; dissolution; separating	*lysis*
	destroy; reduce	*lytic*
macro	large	
mal	bad	
	softening	*malacia*
mamm	breast	
mandibul	mandible	
	madness; insane desire	*mania*
mast	breast	

Prefix	Definition	Suffix
mastoid	mastoid	
maxill	maxilla	
meat	meatus (opening)	
	enlargement	*megaly*
melan	black	
men	menstruation	
mening	meninges	
menisc	meniscus	
ment	mind	
meso	middle	
meta	after; beyond; change	
	instrument used to measure	*meter*
metr	uterus	
	measurement	*metry*
micro	small	
mon	one	
morph	form; shape	*morph*
muc	mucus	
multi	many	
my	muscle	
myc	fungus	
myel	bone marrow; spinal cord	
myelon	bone marrow	
myo	muscle	
myring	eardrum	
narc	stupor	
nas	nose	

Prefix	Definition	Suffix
nat	birth	
necr	death (cells; body)	
neo	new	
nephr	kidney	
neuro	nervous system	
noct	night	
nulli	none	
nyct	night	
	night	nyctal
ocul	eye	
	smell	odia
	pain	odynia
	radiographic imaging	ography
	resembling	oid
olig	scanty; few	
	one who studies/practises; specialist	ologist
	the science of; study of	ology
	tumour; swelling	oma
omphal	umbilicus; navel	
onc	tumour	
onych	nail	
oo	egg; ovum	
oophor	ovary	
	rapid flow of blood	oorhagia
ophth	eye	
ophthalm	eye	
	vision; condition	opia
	to projection	opsy

Prefix	Definition	Suffix
opt	vision	
or	mouth	
orch	testis; testicle	
orchi	testis; testicle	
orchid	testis; testicle	
organ	organ	
	suturing; repairing	*orrhaphy*
	flow; excessive discharge	*orrhoea*
	rupture	*orrhexis*
orth	straight	
	referring to	*ory*
	visualisation using endoscope	*oscopy*
	abnormal condition; increased	*osis*
oste	bone	
	creation of an artificial opening	*ostomy*
ot	ear	
	incision for the removal of	*otomy*
	pertaining to	*ous*
ov	egg	
ox	oxygen	
	oxygen	*oxia*
pachy	thick	
paed	child	
palat	palate	
pan	all; total	
pancreat	pancreas	
papill	nipple	
par	bear; give birth to; labour	

SECTION

5

Prefix	Definition	Suffix
para	beside; beyond; around	
parathyroid	parathyroid gland	
	slight paralysis	paresis
part	bear; give birth to; labour	
patell	patella	
path	disease	path
	disease	pathy
pector	chest	
pelv	pelvis; pelvic bone	
	abnormal reduction in number	penia
	digestion	pepsia
per	through	
peri	surrounding (outer)	
perine	perineum	
peritone	peritoneum	
petr	stone	
	surgical fixation; suspension	pexy
phac	lens of the eye	
phag	eat; swallow	
	eating; swallowing	phagia
phak	lens of the eye	
phalang	finger	
pharang	pharynx	
phas	speech	
	love	philia
	love	phily

Prefix	Definition	Suffix
phleb	vein	
	abnormal fear of; aversion to	*phobia*
	sound; voice	*phonia*
	feeling	*phoria*
phot	light	
phren	mind	
physi	nature	
	growth	*physis*
	formation; development; a growth	*plasia*
plasm	plasma	
	growth; substance; formation	*plasm*
	plastic or surgical repair	*plasty*
	paralysis	*plegia*
pleur	pleura	
	breathing	*pnea*
pneum	lung; air	
pneumat	lung; air	
pneumon	lung; air	
pod	foot	
	formation	*poiesis*
poikil	varied; irregular	
poli	grey matter	
poly	many; much	
polyp	polyp; small growth	
	passage	*porosis*
post	after; posterior	
	meal	*prandial*

Prefix	Definition	Suffix
pre	before; in front of	
prim	first	
pro	before	
proct	rectum	
prostat	prostate gland	
proximal	nearest to the centre	
pseud	fake; false	
psych	mind	
	dropping; sagging; prolapse	*ptosis*
	spitting	*ptysis*
pub	pubis	
puerper	childbirth	
pulmon	lung	
pupill	pupil	
py	pus	
pyel	renal pelvis	
pylor	pylorus (pyloric sphincter)	
pyr	fever; heat	
quadr	four	
rachi	vertebra; spinal/vertebral column	
radi	radius	
radic	nerve root	
radicul	nerve root	
re	back	
rect	rectum	
renal	kidney	
retin	retina	
retro	back; behind	

Prefix	Definition	Suffix
rhabd	rod-shaped, striated	
rhin	nose	
rhiz	nerve root	
rhytid	wrinkles	
	excessive flow	*rrhagia*
	discharge	*rrhoea*
salp	fallopian (uterine) tube	
	fallopian tube	*salpinx*
sarc	flesh; connective tissue	
	malignant tumour	*sarcoma*
scapul	scapula (shoulder bone)	
	split; fissure	*schisis*
scler	sclera	
	hardening	*sclerosis*
scoli	crooked; curved	
	instrument for visual examination	*scope*
	visual examination	*scopic*
	visual examination	*scopy*
seb	sebum (oil)	
semi	half	
	infection	*sepsis*
sept	septum	
sial	saliva	
sigmoid	sigmoid	
sinus	sinus	
	state of	*sis*
somat	body	
somn	sleep	

APPENDICES

Prefix	Definition	Suffix
son	sound	
	sudden involuntary muscle contraction	*spasm*
sperm	spermatozoon; sperm	
spermat	spermatozoon; sperm	
sphygm	pulse	
spir	breathe; breathing	
splen	spleen	
spondyl	vertebra; spinal/vertebral column	
	contraction	*stalsis*
staped	stapes (middle ear bone)	
staphyl	grapelike clusters	
	control; stop	*stasis*
	constriction; narrowing	*stenosis*
stern	sternum	
steth	chest	
stomat	mouth	
strept	twisted chains	
sub	under; below	
super	over; above	
supra	above	
sym	together; joined	
syn	together; joined	
synovi	synovium; synovial membrane	
system	system	
tachy	fast; rapid	
tars	tarsals; edge of eyelid	

Prefix	Definition	Suffix
ten	tendon	
tend	tendon	
tendin	tendon	
test	testis; testicle	
tetra	four	
therm	heat	
thorac	thorax; chest	
	chest	*thorax*
thromb	clot	
thym	thymus gland	
thyr	thyroid gland	
thyroid	thyroid gland	
tibi	tibia	
	birth; labour	*tocia*
tom	cut; section	
	instrument used to cut	*tome*
ton	tension; pressure	
tonsill	tonsils	
top	place	
	poison	*tox*
toxic	poison	
trache	trachea	
trachel	neck; neck-like	
trans	through; across; beyond	
tri	three	
trich	hair	
	surgical crushing	*tripsy*
	nourishment	*trophy*

Prefix	Definition	Suffix
tympan	eardrum; middle ear	
	little	*ule*
uln	ulna	
ultra	beyond; excess	
ungu	nail	
uni	one	
ur	urine; urinary tract	
	micturition	*uresis*
ureter	ureter	
urethr	urethra	
	urine; urination	*uria*
urin	urine; urinary tract	
uter	uterus	
uvul	uvula	
vagin	vagina	
valv	valve	
valvul	valve	
vas	vessel; duct	
ven	vein	
ventricul	ventricle	
vertebr	vertebra; spinal/vertebral column	
vesic	bladder; sac	
vesicul	seminal vesicles	
viscer	internal organs	
vulv	vulva	
xanth	yellow	
xer	dry	

References

1. Greulich WW, Pyle SI, Waterhouse AM 1971 A radiographic standard of reference for the growing hand and wrist. Case Western Reserve University, Chicago

2. Tanner JM, Whitehouse RH, Cameron N, Marshall WA, Healy MJR, Goldstein H 1983 Assessment of skeletal maturity and prediction of adult height, 2nd edn. Academic Press, London

3. Royal College of Radiologists 2003 Making the best use of a Department of Clinical Radiology. Guidelines for doctors, 5th edn. Royal College of Radiologists, London

4. National Radiological Protection Board 1994 Guidelines on radiology standards in primary dental care. NRPB, Oxford

5. National Radiological Protection Board and the Department of Health 2001 Guidance notes for dental practitioners on the safe use of x-ray equipment. NRPB, Oxford. Available online: www.hpa.org.uk/radiation/publications/misc_ publications/dental_guidance_notes.pdf

6. Royal College of Radiologists 2005 Standards for iodinated intravascular contrast agent administration to adult patients. Royal College of Radiologists, London

7. Royal College of Radiologists 1996 Advice on the management of reactions to intravenous contrast media. Royal College of Radiologists, London

Bibliography

Ballinger PW, Frank ED 2003 Pocket guide to radiography, 5th edn. Mosby, St Louis

Ballinger PW, Frank ED, Merrill V 2003 Merrill's atlas of radiographic positions and radiologic procedures, 10th edn. Mosby, London

Bontrager KL, Lampignano JP 2005 Textbook of radiographic positioning and related anatomy, 6th edn. Mosby, Philadelphia

British Society of Paediatric Radiology 2007 Standard for skeletal surveys in suspected non-accidental injury (NAI) in children. Available online: www.bspr.org.uk/nai.htm

Bull S 2005 Skeletal radiography. A concise introduction to projection radiography. Toolkit Publications, Stanley

Carver E, Carver B 2006 Medical imaging techniques, reflection and evaluation. Churchill Livingstone, London

Chapman S, Nakielny R 2001 A guide to radiological procedures, 4th edn. WB Saunders, Edinburgh

College of Radiographers 2000 The Ionising Radiation (Medical Exposure) Regulations 2000. Guidance for radiographers. College of Radiographers, London

Dawson P, Cosgrove DO, Grainger RG 1999 Textbook of contrast media. ISIS Medical Media, Oxford

Eisenberg RL, Dennis CA, May CR 1995 Radiographic positioning, 2nd edn. Little, Brown, London

Ellis H, Logan BM, Dixon AK 2001 Human sectional anatomy. Pocket atlas of body sections, CT and MRI images, 2nd edn. Arnold, London

Hart D, Wall BF 2002 Radiation exposure of the UK population from medical and dental x-ray examinations. National Radiological Protection Board, Chilton

Moses KP, Banks JC, Nava PB, Petersen D 2005 Atlas of clinical gross anatomy. Mosby, Philadelphia

National Radiological Protection Board 1993 Board statement on diagnostic medical exposures to ionizing radiation during pregnancy and estimates of late radiation risks to the UK population. Documents of the NRPB 4 4 1-14. NRPB, London

Sutherland R (ed) 2003 Pocketbook of radiographic positioning, 2nd edn. Churchill Livingstone, Edinburgh

Whitley AS, Alsop CW, Moore AD (eds) 1999 Clark's special procedures in diagnostic imaging. Butterworth-Heinemann, Oxford

Whitley AS, Sloane C, Hoadley G, Moore AD, Alsop CW (eds) 2005 Clark's positioning in radiography, 12th edn. Hodder Arnold, London